Timely, compelling, extraordinary must read!
And add the landing-page-website here

"This is a courageous guide book that will appeal to all who long to connect to their own inner sources of power and healing. Bless yourself and follow Andrea's daring and successful trek on the healing path."

Betina Lindsey, Author and Writer
Shamanic Practitioner
Sound Healing Therapist
Founding Director, Zion Canyon Native Flute School in Southern Utah

"Andrea's eclectic approach to healing is unique and effective. She has been instrumental in my own spiritual and psychological growth and I attribute a large part of my personal expansion to my work with her. I encourage you to read this book so that you too can achieve the happiness and peace you seek."

Patricia Duley, M.D.
Board Certified Internal Medicine
Certified Primordial Sound Meditation Instructor

"I have worked with Andrea in addressing some highly challenging circumstances in my life the past two years. Her compassion, caring and insights have been incredibly helpful. I have gained clarity and peace as a result of her assistance and direction. Andrea has distilled a large body of healing practices and traditions allowing a practical and highly efficient process for growth and transformation. Her wisdom and teachings are a true blessing."

Mike Zimburean, M.D., Psychiatrist
Private Practice, Mill Creek, WA

"Andrea uses her extraordinary gifts of vision and clarity to elevate all those who know in their hearts they can enhance their existence."

Tom Belli
Teacher of Science of Creative Intelligence
CEO of No Worries Consulting

"I attended Andrea's Extraordinary Health Retreat at Omega Institute last fall. It turned out to be the most transformative week of my life. I trudged there missing a piece of my soul that had died along with my brother. A few days later, I happily skipped away from the Omega Campus - a healed person. Almost a year later, my body and soul continue to heal and I believe I am in "Extraordinary Health" thanks to my healer, my friend - Andrea Becky Hanson"

Jean Daniello
Merging Rivers Healing Retreats, Assistant to Director
COO of No Worries Consulting
Documentary Screen Writer

"Andrea Becky Hanson is a wise, experienced guide to the ways of the spirit. Light Through the Keyhole is a marvelous compendium of techniques that show you how to increase your mental and physical energy and develop the awareness to navigate life's challenges as you access the realm of infinite possibility.

Among the many methods described is the Kundalini yoga meditation for Addiction, which is a powerfully effective way to de-magnetize your brain's interlock with any addictive substance or negative behavioral pattern. Major results can occur with a practice of three minutes a day.

Light Through the Keyhole will be a valuable resource for many people."

Harijiwan, Kundalini Teacher and Teacher Trainer

Light Through The Keyhole

Unlock Your Joy
In This World of Relentless Stress

BEST KEPT SECRETS OF EXTRAORDINARY

HOLISTIC ENERGY HEALING

ANDREA BECKY HANSON

Published by Motivational Press, Inc.
2360 Corporate Circle
Suite 400
Henderson, NV 89074
www.MotivationalPress.com

Manufactured in the United States of America.

ISBN: 978-1-62865-015-0

Publishing Date: September 10, 2013
Edition Number: 1st Edition

It is in deepest gratitude, I dedicate this book to each person, animal, spirit and aspect of nature I have encountered in my life. For each has either knowingly or unknowingly helped me, taught me, guided me, and reminded me who I am, why I am here and what I care about. Also to the kind, gentle and powerful Divine Creator who enabled these encounters and gave me the ability to experience and to choose, and who offered me free will and freed my will with understanding, compassion, forgiveness, love and the opportunity to share what I have learned. I am infinitely grateful to all.

Sat Nam,

Andrea Becky

Dear Reader,

In this new world of relentless challenges, it is necessary for me to explain that the information about holistic and energy healing methods and technologies mentioned, explained or recommended in *Light Through the Keyhole*, are not meant to be a substitute for medical advice or treatment. Also, the benefits and results experienced by me and/or others mentioned in this writing are personal, single-study descriptions, and your benefits and results will, of course, vary. I am also obligated to say that I and/or the publisher are not and cannot be responsible for any consequences incurred by the use of the information or modalities mentioned in this book. In other words, I cannot legally or ethically promise that you will receive specific benefit and/or healing from what is intended and offered in this book. The irony of this disclaimer is that each of us is ultimately responsible for our own health and well-being!

As you read through the book, I believe you will see that the intent and passion in the message becomes obvious. Over time it has been made clear to me through tradition, all kinds of messages, and most of all from the loud voices of my heart and soul that I must pass forward my experiences. For this reason, I share my revelations, realizations, and resolutions with whomever is interested and may benefit. All the cases and studies and stories included in *Light Through the Keyhole* are true and involve real people (and animals) whose names have been changed in some circumstances to protect their privacy.

Finally, I am grateful for whatever forces put this book in your hands. I treasure and welcome your time, attention and interest in seeking understanding, extraordinary health and an exquisitely joyous life, for that is truly our individual and collective birthright.

Sat Nam,

Andrea Becky

Andrea Becky Hanson

Light Through the Keyhole

My longing, seeking and searching
Led me to the door of self discovery once again
The door still, in my mind, locked to me
With key in hand
The light through the keyhole blinded me
As I dared to approach
Self doubt and fear warned me to stop
A stronger sense of desolation pushed me closer this time
The door was not locked and swung open freely
I gasped at the sameness on the other side
Except for the mirror reflecting the light within me...
My heart filled with understanding and
I wept and laughed recalling all the years
I believed I was just on the wrong side of the door
And that the light was only somewhere outside of me

Andrea Becky - 11/11/11

Table of Contents

Table of Contents

Table of Contents

Introduction

The choice to live fully and joyfully is in each everyday endeavor.

Andrea Becky

The small cement step that separated the driveway from my mother's flower garden was a perfect perch for me and my dog, Molly. I had just planted the seeds Mrs. Schmidt, the nice lady who lived across the street, had given me the day before. I was admiring my work and loving the feel and the smell of the rich moist earth and wondering if the seeds would sprout today. I was three years old.

I planted the seeds near my favorite tree I called the yellow chain tree, which was in bloom and was much older than I, but only as tall as my twelve year-old brother. Molly barked and I looked up to see Mr. Bjork pulling in his driveway. I wondered why he went so slow and opened his garage doors, put his car in his garage, and closed the doors every time whether he was home for a few minutes or for a long time. I wondered about a lot of things. Why do we live here and not somewhere else? How did we get here? Where did Molly come from? Why do people do the same things every day even if they don't like them? Why do you have to be five before you can go to school, and why does school start at 9 o'clock? Why do people talk about the same things every day? And why don't they ever talk about some things?

Mom came to the side door of the house across the driveway from where I was sitting, and said,

"Becky", (My childhood name) "Where is the good scissors?" I automatically closed my eyes just for a moment and saw them on a stepping stone in the back yard. I told Mom where they were and she came out of the house and went to the back gate and into the back yard. She came back with the scissors in her hand and said,

"You know when you use the scissors to put them back where they belong."

"I didn't use them," I said.

"Well then," Mom said, "how did you know where they were?

"I just know," I said.

"Now don't lie and make it worse Pevekka," (my name in Greek which she would use when reprimanding me) and she went back in the house.

I thought nothing of the fact I could see lost things, but I somehow did get in trouble for that. Also, my older brother and sister didn't mind at all if I took the blame for misplaced things and would never admit to their part in it. I also knew the cousins were coming over to play before they got there. My mom said it was just my dreams coming true. I guess that made sense because I really liked my cousins. We would all climb trees and play with my imaginary friends, and we would eat the ripe cherries from the big cherry tree.

As you may have guessed by now, I was "one of those kids" that have a lot of imaginary friends. They would play anything I wanted, any time I wanted; they were great fun and never really wanted or needed anything else. It didn't really occur to me that I was "different," but I did learn to be quiet more often than not when I knew something no one else seemed to know.

It didn't seem strange to me that my father was not there. He died in a car accident right before my first birthday. All I remember is everyone crying real loud, and going to my aunt's house in the dark... and the crib I was in... and the trees outside the window, and how they always wrapped me too tight with the blanket and everyone was sad and I felt left out. Mother called me in for lunch.

Although we were a family of very modest means, especially after my father left, Mother always made it seem we were wealthy by providing fresh wholesome delicious food, sewing wonderful clothes for us, keeping a clean orderly house, music and flowers and great books, vegetables from the garden, and a loving environment with honor, direction and purpose.

When I recall my early years, I can feel the blissful innocent state of wonderment and awe. I can remember it was without judgment, disapproval or thinking it should be different or I should be different. There was an atmosphere of a complete sense of safety, interrelatedness, freedom and being able to spontaneously, authentically and honestly express myself, my curiosity and desires and share with others. This book is about the journey from that blissful state and self-image. The loss and the rediscovery of it, and what I learned along the way...how it all unfolded for me, and how and why it can unfold for you as well into your joyous life.

Section One

Getting Started

New Living Skills for Our New World

Our Already New World

> *At times we must jump first and build our*
> *wings on the way down.*

> -Thich Nhat Hanh

I have to smile a little when I hear someone say that there will be great change and the world will not be the same as we now know it. In my experience, the world is now not as we have ever known it and has not been for some time. The recent rate and amount of dramatic change and evolution on all levels in our lives is so accelerated, our normal learning, coping and adapting abilities have been intensely challenged. Our need to learn and apply new skills and understandings has become heightened and, some argue, imperative for survival, let alone for a joyous life. We have a learning curve that is not only straight up but bends over backwards a bit and sometimes seems to go back to square one.

The good news is all that we need to learn and adapt is available and accessible to us right now. If what you desire seems to elude you, it is most likely because you may not be aware of the new world healing and transformational tools and techniques or how to use them. *Light Through the Keyhole* is about the methods and practices that help you access the knowledge, awareness and experience that will enable you to know who you really are and live the joyous healthy life you desire...without disappointment, struggle and with grace and ease. "Is that really possible?" you might say. And I say..."It is!"

In this section, you will learn some very important foundational skills, concepts and considerations that are necessary for you to know to optimize your journey to your true self and the joyous life that is actually your birthright.

Throughout this section, there will be opportunities introduced to practice the new skills and concepts. They are samples of healing practices. They are called healing practices because when doing them, you are practicing healing...actually, you are healing.

The Belief Gap - That is Unbelievable!

A belief is not merely an idea that the mind possesses;
it is an idea that possesses the mind.

-Robert Bolton

The *Belief Gap* is a phenomenon that exists from our natural propensity to want to safely believe what we believe within the range of our perceived reality. We are occupied with our lives and responsibilities and pursuits, and in most cases doing a pretty good job of making it through. When an idea or suggestion or experience comes into our awareness that is far from our everyday reality, we have no way of believing it could possibly be true because we have no point of reference. An example of this is the statement, "live *a joyous life without disappointment, struggle and with grace and ease."* If that has not been our experience, our normal reaction is that it's a nice thought, but absurd, not possible and/or in some cases... some kind of subversive crazy notion, and usually we will dismiss it. Our beliefs result from our everyday experiences and learning, and many are conscious, and many are sub-conscious. They form the foundation of our thoughts and actions.

I predict and expect you will experience the belief gap phenomenon several times when reading this book. The new and ancient healing therapies and technologies and the multicultural and multidimensional nature of this material, as well as the original methods offered, will most likely be somewhat foreign to you. No worries, however, because it is all based on universal principles, and some part of you will sense, know and experience the truth in it.

Felt Sense - Knowing Beyond Knowing

All phenomena exist for us only when we pay attention to them.
Attention brings out hidden secrets.

-Buddha

A first step towards expanding your knowledge, awareness and experience is to know that much of what you need or want to know is at a level beyond the five senses and rational thought. It is from an unseen field of energy and information and is a source of wisdom which is expressed and accessed through feeling or sensation. By putting attention on what we sometimes call intuition, a hunch, or a "just a feeling," information can be gained and solutions, shifts in perception and new knowledge can result. This is a practice of paying attention to having a sense of something long enough to garner what the message actually is. Just this awareness will change the way you treat this *felt sense*. As you gain more self trust in this body awareness, the *felt sense* information garnered will assist you in your thoughts, choices and actions. The term "Felt Sense" was coined by Eugene T. Gendlin, Ph.D in his 1978 book, *Focusing*, which is a good source for understanding this concept in depth.

The Eternal Now Moment - It All Happens Right Here

Nothing ever happened in the past; it happened in the Now.
Nothing will ever happen in the future; it will happen in the Now.

-Eckhart Tolle

Now is where we live. Now is the only time in which we have the time and power to create. Everything originates in the now moment. Eckhart Tolle in his book, *The Power of Now*, explores "The Now" fully, and recommends making it the primary focus of your life. The problem is that it is more difficult than it sounds. The powerful life-giving Now moment can be easily missed, forgotten and wasted with attention on the past or the future and the distractions in the now, or it can be fully lived and called upon at any moment. We know we are in The Now when we sense the eternal, infinite, timeless nature of it.

The Now Opportunity – Insurance

It was too soon. It was too late. Now the now is past and has changed our fate....

-Andrea Becky

Have you ever noticed that if you act on something at the earliest possible opportunity, it happens quickly and effortlessly? And what happens if you flag it, put it on a shelf, on a to-do list or in a file for later? Most of the time, it is more difficult to do, if in fact you actually get to it, and/or it will be postponed further. Do you ever move things from yesterday's to-do list to today's?

Since now is the only real time we have to learn, live and create, throughout the book we will pause to experience what is being discussed using various healing practices in the moment. These are called "now opportunities" for application of what you learn and coined and identified as the *NowOpp@(Concept).*

NowOpps will provide a practical flow of experiential learning while you are in the flow of the energy and information of the subject or concept. The energy in which the information is presented will assist your deeper learning and understanding and will insure and deepen the energetic learning experience. This increases the odds that you will embody the concept energetically.

NowOpp@NowMoment

Be seated comfortably and close your eyes. Take one or two deep breaths and relax. For two to three minutes, simply contemplate the nature of "The Now." Attempt to find the beginning, middle and end of it, get a felt sense of it and develop a new perception of it. Take another deep breath when you feel complete.

The Quintessential Life Determining Choice Point

The choice to live fully and joyfully lives within each everyday endeavor.

-Andrea Becky

The Now moment is the home of the "Choice Point," that critical instant when we choose, consciously or unconsciously, what we do, think, or say in that moment and line up for the consequences. That instant shapes us, our lives and how we relate to everything around us and our future. A *Choice Point* is the counter point of a "Trigger." It gives us time to actually choose, rather than react.

The Now moment is all the time we need for spontaneous right choice and right action if we stay connected and know who we are and why we are here...that is a big "IF." I can remember when I was first learning to meditate and introduced to the concept of living in the present moment. My belief gap said, "You will go crazy if you have to be aware of making a choice in every moment. That's impossible! You only make a choice occasionally when you need to or want to." What I know now is those thoughts were a function of my rational mind and my ego that had been running my life, and doing a pretty good job, and did not have the ability to fathom being in a state of potentiality and choice in each moment. I didn't know learning to meditate would change all that... more about that later, but right now here is an introduction to the power of the *Choice Point* at home in *The Now:*

NowOpp@ChoicePoint

Be comfortably seated. Take one or two deep breaths and relax. Close your eyes and take two to three minutes to experience the energy of the *Choice Point*, that moment of choice that changes everything. Practice choosing repeatedly in the eternal now moment. For example, in the essence of the now, choose something you want more of in your life, like love, abundance, great health or joy. You will notice that the words "I want" won't work. Now time choice point application requires present tense or being. So it's not "I want joy" it is "I choose joy," or "I am joy." Enjoy! And be aware of the *Felt Sense* during this exercise.

Grounding and Centering

> *We do not see things as they are; we see them as we are.*
>
> -The Talmud

As we will learn in the next section of the book, we are a field of energy within the universal, unified field of energy. It is important to be centered and grounded as a spirit in a physical body when on

6

the earth plane. That is our optimum position to experience joy, tranquility, fulfillment and awareness, and to live life's joys and challenges in the best way. This will be expanded upon in other parts of the book as needed. For now, I would like to create an opportunity to get a sense of what it feels like to consciously ground and center so we can move on in that state.

NowOpp@GroundedAndCentered

Take a moment and direct your attention inward and take note of how you feel. Take a couple of deep breaths and relax. Close your eyes and put your hands on your thighs palms down. Now imagine you are rooted to the earth just like a big oak tree with deep, strong roots and feel the support and nurturing sense of that image. Now at the same time, imagine your energy fully uplifted to the heavens forming a connection with all that is. Feel yourself totally connected, balanced and centered within yourself. Notice any subtle sensations you feel. Put your attention on your breath and feel the power of being grounded and centered. Take one or two deep breaths, slowly open your eyes and note how you feel now.

De-Stressing from 21st Century Stress Epidemic Can Be Distressing!

The particular challenge we have in this era of human evolution is the incredible fast pace and 24/7/366 constancy with which new information and energy becomes available to us, and the incredible speed it is transmitted and downloaded. In fact, media experts tell us the amount of information available to us in the last three years is more than the information available in the last 6,000 years all together. The effects of this shift in our environment are prevalent because in most cases, our learned coping mechanisms and our nervous systems are not quite up to the task of taking in and processing the incredible amount of information we seek and/or are exposed to.

In some circles, high stress is actually considered a mark of an important person and in many cases the belief gap possibilities have increased exponentially and our minds simply do not know what to do with all the energy and information, new beliefs and ways of doing things.

These circumstances decrease our natural abilities to handle stress because we tend to remain in a constant state of activity in an attempt to deal with the stress. Because the natural living and healing cycle of all living things is alternating activity and rest. Under stress, we are in a constant state of activity and/or not living in harmony with the natural cycle of all living things, and our bodies are not able to heal and rejuvenate as they were designed to. And, our natural healing abilities become suppressed.

Today, there is an increase of emerging and chronic disorders and diseases. Some are identified as 21st century epidemics. They are named and coded regularly to diagnose, describe and identify the depth and seriousness of maladies such as, Relentless Stress Syndrome, Post Traumatic Stress, Adrenal Fatigue, Cold Depression and all kinds of complex anxiety, depression, cancer, immune system deficiencies, and mental-emotional and personality disorders to name a few.

There is plenty of research to show that there is a direct correlation between continual stress and disease. Stress syndromes and disorders are prevalent and numerous and well-noted in the allopathic medical and psychological manuals, journals and research. There are endless categories noted with specific causes and symptoms. It is referred to in some cases as "the invisible injury." Possible treatments range from none to rehabilitation methods, pharmaceutical, psychiatric interventions, hospitalization and perhaps institutionalization depending on severity of symptoms.

In holistic diagnosis, stress is considered the first phase of disease and taken very seriously before it transforms or transmutes into even more serious stages of illness. Since the holistic approach is to pursue dynamic balance, release interruptions in the energy system, and reinstate natural cycles, all treatment is focused on those goals as early in the detection process as possible and much attention is put on prevention. The symptoms are the clues to imbalance, but the holistic focus is the original source of the problem and the restoration of health of the whole being.

The holistic, body-centered, energetic approaches and practices of entraining with natural cycles are considered the New Medicine. Even though they are based on ancient wisdom, they are supported by the leading edge scientific findings and are incredibly empowering and effective. The ancient technologies and leading edge therapies and scientific findings are understandable and offer empowering paths through the immense and innumerable challenges of our times.

Light Through the Keyhole is about discovering the keys you possess right now that will unlock your understanding and experience, assist you safely on your path and close the gap that keeps you from your desired life. This holistic energetic view of life is focused on healing the sources of negativity and unhappiness to enable the symptoms of stress, struggle, disease and suffering to fall away. It is in this way we become free to live the joyous, fulfilling life we are meant to live!

NowOpp@ActivityAndRestCycle

5 - 5 – ? Breath is used to signal your brain that you are safe and stimulates the relaxation response. When we are stressed or suffering from unfound fear or anxiety or just plain nervous, we tend to hold our breath on the inhale. This signals the brain we are in danger and the brain prepares the body for attack. When the danger is not actually real, we can signal the brain that we are safe and it will begin to prepare us for safety and the symptoms of anxiety will subside. Be comfortably seated and take three full breaths and relax. Inhale slowly and deeply to a slow count of five (about a second each if possible). Immediately exhale slowly and completely to a slow count of five (same length as inhale). Hold and rest in the space at the end of the exhale for 3 - 5 long counts or as long as it feels good. Notice all sensations as part of your experience. Continue for at least two minutes or until feeling calm and balanced. Count can be increased to 7 -7 -? or 10 -10 - ? as long as it is comfortable and as you increase your ability to consciously control your breath and calm your physiology.

Matrix Learning for Sustainable Awareness and Understanding

I did not arrive at my understanding of the universe through my rational mind

-Albert Einstein

The concepts, ideas and processes in this book are presented and intended to be what I call a "matrix learning experience." This includes the familiar, natural ways of learning, such as rational, factual, deductive and informational. However, felt sense, creative thinking, conscious day-dreaming, visualizing and imaging are all emphasized, as well. There is also a good dose of exploring the formerly unknown and "not-having-to-know-the-outcome" experiential learning, too. We are in a new amazing age of energy and information in which the ability to learn in many different ways is necessary for our evolution, and some argue, our survival.

"Matrix learning" is different from pure rational, deductive thought in that understanding comes in where allowed and not necessarily in logical, numerical or outline order. It fills in like a digital screen and eventually makes meaningful sense we can identify that enables us to shift our perception and understanding. In this way, we expand our ability to seek knowledge in an abstract subtle way that serves us in the physical world and in our quickly expanding virtual world. It is like connecting the dots in a virtual, multidimensional way as your conscious awareness expands.

Holistic energy healing takes place at the most subtle vibrational level of our being as it increases and expands our level of consciousness and conscious awareness. This healing is detectable immediately by the sense of a higher level of well-being; by the way the world seems like a better place to us; how our life flows more freely; how our communication and relationships improve; and how our desires are met more readily. These changes are sustainable and not random as you may previously have experienced. Sometimes it seems these changes are miracles after years of failed attempts to change your life significantly. Just the explanation of this approach may be uncomfortable for you and trigger your belief gap. This will be especially true if you are particularly intellectual in your orientation. The process was frustrating to me in the beginning, but I have discovered the benefits and gifts of expanding our abilities to learn in many ways are innumerable and required for a truly authentic and joyous life. So, I invite you to join this unprecedented adventure in self-knowledge and revelation. It will take dedication and willingness to use your creative mind more for solutions to problems and periods of not having to know the outcome in the moment...

On Not Having to Know - A Skill that Goes with Matrix Learning

...go slowly, smile and breathe...

-Tich Nhat Han

It was a pleasant room, lovingly decorated, and with many people who were in the energy of hope. I could feel trepidation, determination and a feint feeling of instability in the air. I didn't feel I belonged there because the wedge of denial kept me isolated in my disbelief that my daughter, KiKi, could really be addicted to anything. On the information table, were some hand drawn postcards that depicted a happy girl in a flower garden and said, "Happiness is not having to know." This caught and held my attention as my mind scanned my experiences and tried to find meaning with no success. I picked up one of the cards and put it in my purse to contemplate it later. Each guest of honor announced their respective birthday of sobriety and received their token of success and applause and hugs and kisses of celebration. I was still puzzled by the mixed atmosphere of joy and fear and not aware enough of my own feelings to know that that was within me, too. We were pleased that KiKi had completed the 30-day program, and was celebrating her 30-day sobriety and was coming home with us today. I was busy trying to understand the language of addiction and recovery and trying to make sense of it and the party festivities went by quickly. When all the thank you's and goodbye's and name and phone number exchanges tapered off, we left together to go home. On the way to the car, KiKi said she wanted to drive. Her dad said no, her brother shook his head, and we were in the combative family dynamic less than five minutes from leaving the facility. Everyone got in the car in a thick silence and we proceeded to the freeway home. On the way, I pulled out the postcard that still had some of my attention and asked everyone if they knew what this meant. The tense silence was not a fruitful ground for answers, ideas or suggestions. It would be 15 years before I really understood what "Happiness is not having to know" meant. What I knew at that time was only that the thought helped someone get over something, and having to know leads you down a rabbit hole.

When Too Much Is Not Enough

Just as you have the impulse to do something...stop.

-Anonymous Early Zen Scripture

Repeating and/or addictive self-destructive thoughts, behaviors and actions are never about the substances, activities or behaviors we think they are. They relate back to faulty self-knowledge and self-image. A very high majority of people I know and have consulted with about looking for healing from addiction relate that they feel lost and don't know who they are anymore. They nearly always say that they were trying to find themselves and meaning and purpose for their existence. The obvious error, of course, is looking outside one's self for identity and meaning. Success is only derived from directing the search within, not to what we think we know about ourselves, but to what we do not yet know. That is the tricky part, and often, a pitfall on the path to wholeness. The good news is that correct self-image and true identity and purpose are addressed in detail throughout this book.

Denial – How Do We Know What We Don't Know?

Guilt and fear are the guardians of denial.

-Andrea Becky

We are pretty good at finding out about the bad things we think, say or do by feeling the detrimental effects and/or being called out about it. However, the real problem is realizing the real truth of who we really are. The denial of our greatness, limitlessness, perfection and self-healing nature plagues us, and we don't even know it...until it doesn't any more. The fear that we are actually worse than the flawed person we think we are can keep us from discovering our true amazing potential. This is the book that can resolve this web of misunderstanding and misinterpretation of our true identity and purpose. Good choice!

The Four Doors to a Joyous, Healthy Life

You can't do something you don't know,
if you keep on doing what you do know.

-F.M. Alexander

How do we create sustained transformation, extraordinary health and a joyous life?

We are all familiar with change...temporary change, inability to change, cataclysmic change and how some things never change. What this book is about is transformation, actually transmutation or permanent change that literally gives us a new reality where the old reality seems like another lifetime and no longer has a hold on us.

We already live in a world where perception and reality change rapidly, and we are in the process of adapting and evolving to live well in that new world. The holistic energy approach to transformation and healing offers the ability to transform completely without struggle and with grace and ease. More good news is that the latest scientific findings, particularly about the brain, the nervous systems and our true physical nature, support the ancient healing premises and processes of transformation and enlightenment. I have found the process of evolving on all levels to be a natural matter of time and life cycles, but also a matter of consciously following some repeating pathways, generally in this sequence: acquiring knowledge, opening awareness and understanding through experience. This pathway results in the realizing of a new dimension of personal orientation, thinking and actions and experiences.

An example of this is the experience of becoming ill...you are well, you have signs of becoming ill, you become ill, you might even say, "I can't believe I am so sick" and you think you will never feel good again. Then at some point you realize you are well and cannot remember the moment you got better, but you are. I believe this "missing moment" is largely a result of our perception-determined reality...we have a perception and beliefs that go along with it, and we act on that premise. Then, our perception changes and we have a new belief and we take different actions in the new reality. And this process repeats. We usually do not change our beliefs without an experience or conflicting new perception that changes our current perception. A classic example of this shift in reality is the ancient belief that the world was flat, and the new experiences, information and perceptions that changed that, prompted different beliefs and actions and created our new reality that the earth is round. Our previous ideas about evolution have been more or less about a passive, long-term process. The current era is demanding a conscious accelerated ability to evolve and adapt intentionally on all levels of being quick. This new evolved, elevated and expanded conscious awareness and way of being is attainable and sustainable through holistic practices and energy healing. I call this holistic evolution, when we are consciously evolving on all levels of our being: physically, intellectually, emotionally, spiritually, socially, culturally, environmentally, and actually globally and galactically.

NowOpp@CreatingAJoyousLife

With this suggested process of holistic evolution in mind, from your current point of view and thinking, please familiarize yourself with the four doors described below. Contemplate the different qualities of the subcategories as you recall personal examples from your life of each category. This will enhance your personal understanding of this process of transformation and personal holistic evolution as we unlock and open these doors on our journey throughout the book.

1. **<u>Door of Knowledge</u>**

   What you need to know, to know what you don't know -

   Knowledge you are born with or into and are taught or assume
   Knowledge gained from seeking your heart's desires, or not
   Knowledge that expands your awareness – beyond right and
   wrong

2. **<u>Door of Awareness</u>**

   The unfolding of questions you do not yet know to ask -

   Awareness of practical everyday living
   Awareness of the heart's desires and/or disappointments
   Awareness from knowledge that changes your awareness

3. **<u>Door of Experience</u>**

   Feeling the truth that changes your truth -

   Experiences that everyone agrees on and you come to expect
   Experiences from seeking the heart's desires, or not
   Experience beyond your accepted or expected reality that
     changes your reality

4. **<u>Door of Transformation</u>**

   Living authentically with grace and ease -

   Transformation of perception and reality bringing
     synchronicity, meaning and miracles
   Transformation bringing being beyond right and wrong and the
     resolution of opposites
   Transformation of wholeness and having no more questions

Section Two

Holistically Speaking

What is Holistic Energy Healing Anyway?!

The holistic approach to healing is based on the knowledge and understanding that nothing is separate and the parts of an organism are inextricably interconnected and only explainable in reference to each other and to the whole organism. Holistic treatment is characterized by treatment regarding the whole being taking into account all levels of being: physical, mental, emotional, spiritual, social and environmental. Symptoms are only indications of an imbalance of parts affecting the whole person. The focus of treatment is towards the origin of the imbalance and treatment is for all aspects of the being. The attitude towards health is not just the absence of disease, but living holistically means adjusting all aspects of your life to maintain the natural dynamic balance of optimum health and well-being.

Energy Healing works on the premise that we are multidimensional, complex fields of vibration, energy, light and information. We are dynamically balanced, harmonic and healthy. The main discovery premise of Energy Healing is: **Any discomfort or disease or stress is due to interruption in our energy field which obstructs the correct flow of energy.** Holistic energy healing treatment may be sought based on symptoms, but treatment focus is on the origin of any discomfort, disorder or disease to restore our natural balance and flow of energy. These concepts will be fully explored and explained throughout the book as will the methods, therapies and technologies to maintain natural balance and flow of energy.

For the time being, in the interest of foundational comparative understanding, please consider the chart on the next page. It includes the roots of major medical systems of healing, their origins, concepts and aspects in a historical context with a very brief etiological map. In addition, there is a categorical explanation of the many holistic healing possibilities available to us now for our healing and evolution.

From one perspective, there are as many paths to healing as there are those who seek healing. As Alice said in *Alice in Wonderland*, "If you don't know where you are going, any path will take you there." What I have found to be a basic experience from seeking knowledge and understanding is the more you gather new challenging information, the more you consciously expand awareness. Then healing, synchronicity, miracles and blessings seem less random. Also,

18

the better your map, the more enjoyable, productive and fulfilling your journey. For me, discovering and navigating the many pathways to health and healing has been quite an adventure and, I will say, not without caution and/or blind faith at times.

What is possible in terms of new integrated health and healing is infinite. What is available for you personally, your family and friends, and your career and/or profession and clients, can be overwhelming. If you choose to help others through healing modalities, the viable paths are many. It is my intention that the following very brief organization of the roots of healing systems and the resulting methods, therapies and techniques will assist you in understanding the focus and differences in the various branches of energy healing. This will begin to serve as a map for your journey through healing.

I know of no complete categorization of healing modalities, and believe most people are most likely unaware of the alternative and integrative categories of healing. Using the following explanations will at least help you know what to put in the search box for further and more detailed and comparative research. It is my hope that this classification will help with your search for understanding.

Aspects of Major Historic Systems of Medicine

Attributes	Ayurvedic Medicine	Chinese Medicine	Greek Medicine	Shamanistic Medicine	Homeopathic Medicine
Origin	India 4000+BC	China 500+BC with roots much earlier	Greece 700+ BC early influence 450 BC major influence Hippocrates	Worldwide Pre-religious practice in Paleolithic Age	Germany 1796
Basic Philosophy	Health depends on an energetic model and is a Science of life - All is one breath (prana) inter-related and maintaining natural dynamic balance with all for optimum health	Health depends on an energetic model - with emphasis on balanced yin and yang energies the four natures integrated anatomical and pathological concepts inner awareness of balance	Health is the absence of disease and based on a biochemical model and following the Hippocratic Oath stating a strict ethical code and scope of practice	Health and healing for disease and disorders lie in dimensions accessed by the initiated practitioner entering other realms and identifying, correcting the causes	Like cures like, and Health depends on the balancing of disease and disorder with minute and sometimes non-molecular (homeopathic) dilutions for a most powerful effect

Aspects of Major Historic Systems of Medicine (*Continued*)

Attributes	Ayurvedic Medicine	Chinese Medicine	Greek Medicine	Shamanistic Medicine	Homeopathic Medicine
Levels of Application	Physical Psychological Emotional Spiritual Environmental	Physical Psychological Environmental	Physical Psychological	Physical, Psychological Emotional Spiritual	Physical Psychological Emotional
Primary Premise	There is a universal inter-related balance that must be maintained. Illness results from imbalance emphasis on prevention and longevity	Illness is interruption of harmonious interaction of inner functional entities and the outside world	By discovering and knowing the categories, symptomology and progression of disease, treatment can be determined	Shaman has power to heal by entering the spirit world for signs, archetypes and answers	All disease is caused by miasma-vapor from decaying or unhealthy substances
Methods of Diagnosis	Detailed and complex questioning and observation of the five senses, posture, habits, pulses, appearance and behavior noting imbalances in the individual mind body constitution	Tracing symptoms to patterns of thought or behavior related to the disharmony by questioning, palpating the pulse and inspecting the tongue	Noting symptoms and through the process of deductive analysis and elimination determining the disorder or disease	Through song, drumming, intuition and as a seer, the Shaman sees the problem and interprets it and through ceremony, archetype, herbs and process, causes the energy to correct	Extensive, holistic, emphasis on individual manifest symptoms or complaints
Methods of Treatment	Information Awareness Experience Yoga Meditation Foods, Herbs, Oils, Nature Purification Massage Aroma Astrology Numerology Surgery Chanting	Prescribed Herbal and animal medicinals, teas and remedies Martial Arts Acupuncture Balancing Qi (Breath) and mind and body	Manipulation of Tissue, Bone, Molecules, Pharmaceutical Surgery, Psychotherapy	Archetypical or animal medicine advice, journey, ceremony and ritual with prescribed substances, articles, fire, water, earth, chanting, keeping a mesa (sacred alter)	Minimum doses of individualized homeopathic remedies
Origin and development of treatment	Largely natural herbs and specific foods and practices	Comprehensive herbal and plant and animal concoctions	Biochemical, plants, synthetic and natural origins	Varies and generally passed down a lineage	Plant, mineral or animal substances repeatedly diluted to a particular strength

In addition to a research tool, this chart is meant to provide a background for methods you may or may not be aware of when seeking the best modalities for your own healing needs.

Although possibilities for healing abound, most people have experienced only one or maybe two healing systems or methods. It was not so long ago that alternative and integrative systems, doctors and practitioners were available only in countries of their origin. Shortly later, they were only available in the United States in a few of the more progressive cities, such as New York and Los Angeles. For a long time, the healing opportunities available to us today were considered "obscured," "not insured" and in some cases, "not real medicine" or "woo-woo" because of the lack of understanding of the basis of holistic energy healing modalities. Hence, the purpose of this chapter is to broaden and widen your awareness of choices, and make you aware of the systems available to you and the fact that many are now insured. This field is changing so fast that by the time you are reading this, it will have changed and evolved even more, but will still provide a basis for information.

This is my analysis having experienced and studied so many of the systems, and my intention was to them categorize in a "functional knowledge" way. Many overlap and belong in multiple categories. Some are better known, cover all aspects of health and are well-developed, and others are a bit more obscure, singular in purpose, but still available options. This is by no means a complete exploration of options, but most certainly an opening to the possibilities, information and as an investigative tool.

The five major healing medical systems were selected based on historic origins, philosophies, and diagnostic and treatment procedures. They are: Ayurvedic, Chinese Medicine, Greek Medicine, Shamanistic and Homeopathic. With this very brief comparative knowledge of the major categories, we can better move on to the exciting evolution of integrated energy healing modalities explained in the next chapter. And now that you are beginning to have an expanded, more correct view of yourself and a better idea of what to expect, you will be able to make your best choices should you choose to seek assistance and healing on any level and/or to expand your healing practice personally or professionally.

Navigating the Multicultural and Multidimensional Roots of Healing

The major healing systems include aspects from the known (physical) to the unknown (theory, intuited knowledge and spiritual realms). There were many inquiries about the common denominator among the systems, and there was consistent agreement that it was a great life force that was universal and indispensible, divine, life-giving and life-sustaining energy. It was a key to open, clear, exploration of all levels of self, all dimensions of the universe, and it was the life force accompanying the breath.

Everything Is Energy and Vibration

We exist ultimately beyond our bodies, minds and spirits and matter in a manifestation of energy and vibration. We didn't build this world...our intentions, learning, awareness and unawareness built it. Our true identity, as Deepak Chopra likes to say, "is not one of human beings having a spiritual experience, but one of spiritual beings having a human experience." This used to be a difficult and foreign concept to embody, particularly in the mechanically-oriented western world.

The ancient rishis and yogis intuited this understanding thousands of years ago and developed detailed intricate healing systems mapping out the body's systems including the energy system for managing the life energy. Chinese Medicine and Indian Ayurvedic Medicine were developed from this understanding. Ancient Shamans and German scientists and doctors understood it was energy that united all things. In Greek medicine, there are many reverences to energy and spirit, however, western medicine developed a differing diagnostic focus and understanding based on symptoms, deductive thinking, pharmacology and manipulation of the body and tissues for treatment.

Ironically now, it is the Quantum Physicists and Neuroscientists whose findings are showing the apparent energy and information life force qualities in matter, and leading the field in the understanding of human behavior, thinking, and healing. And so, Spirituality and Science are merging with the same conclusions about the nature of existence, health and healing. This is a very exciting and evolutionary time and the "Oldknew Medicine" is coming into being.

The Breath as the Divine Life Force

I am That, you are That, all this is That.

-The Veda's

It is undeniable that the breath and life are inseparable and that our physical lives are measured from our fist breath to our last. And of all things, it is the thing that we cannot do without for the shortest period of time and live. However, there are numerous references to the breath as something much more...divine and common among all things, the glue of the universe, a universal flow and vibration, the common connecting energy. Hippocrates spoke of Pneuma, as the vital Force necessary to sustain life and was quoted as saying:

"There is one common flow, one common breathing, all things are in sympathy."

Most of the ancient teachings and healing systems referred to the breath as the source of life or the actual life force and to the energy system that processes the energy of the life force, separate from the respiratory (to re-breathe or inspire) system. Words assigned to describe this force, most of which had spiritual connotations... from the East Indian, Prana; the Chinese, Chi; the Japanese, Qui; the Native Americas, Nature Spirits; the Polynesian, Manna; the Islam, Ru; the Judaic, Rua; the Hawaiian, Ola; the Incan, Kawsay; the Filipino, Karkama; and to the Spanish, Espirito, to mention only a few.

In most eastern cultures, the life force is directly addressed and is generally an everyday awareness of the people. Also, correcting and stimulating the free flow of this vital life source through the energy system and the environment was and is the goal of many healing modalities and a basic understanding in the use of Energy Medicine. The ancient practices of Chinese medicine such as acupuncture are a well-known example of this, as is Feng Shui, the study of energy movement in the environment. Energy Psychology, a leading edge western body of healing methods is also based on this concept.

In the western world, for the most part, the concept of the breath as the life force has remained a physical function which marks the beginning of life and the end of life and to maintain respiration. It is not usually addressed in common health or healing systems, except when referring to breathing and the respiratory system disorders and diseases, and the spiritual and common thread of all living things, aspect of the breath has been somewhat lost. Since it is our most basic healing tool, it will be referred to often in this book and fully explained in Section Four under "Breathing" and Section Six under "Pranayam," the conscious use of the breath.

My Own Pangaea...An Evolution of Understanding Energy Healing Methods, Techniques and Therapies

Many people ask me how I have come to do what I do. My answer is simple...I followed my heart...and soul. I was naturally guided by my intuitive experiences, my mother's naturalist approach to health and life, and studying astrology. As far as I knew, short of playing the Ouija board or telling ghost stories around a campfire, and several obscure healing modalities learned while traveling, most non-traditional practices were something someone else practiced and were either only in books, mystically intuited, passed down through lineages, or in movies. In addition, my traditional education, along with everyone I knew, told me I was a body, mind and with a conscience to consult, and that organized, rational, philosophical and scientific thinking was the sign of brilliance and accomplishment. That belief was culturally and ethnically (being of Greek decent) supported as well, and that was the level of awareness I pursued and entertained. It worked well and was reflected back to me over and over. However, that reality was about to expand and deepen beyond what I could ever have imagined as I followed an inexplicable pushing desire and curiosity to learn the unusual and out of the mainstream thoughts and practices around life and healing modalities.

A Seemingly Insignificant Related Experience

It was 1979, and seven of us had gathered in a modest engaging old home in south San Diego. Each of us was individually drawn for different reasons to the work of Mother Sarita. I had learned of her from a psychokinetic psychic reader our lunch group had gone to a few times, which was very daring for our group. I was the only one in our group who was interested in going to Mother Sarita for this four-session month-long training in an ancient Toltec diagnostic and healing method.

We were standing around a sort of massage table in anticipation of learning the spiritual healing techniques Mother Sarita was famous for...using a raw egg to diagnose problems...and healing through ceremony and prayer. One person, I will call "Tim," had volunteered for the spiritual healing demonstration. We were handed workbooks from which to read along with the copious prayers, in Spanish with a translator who assisted, setting the intention, permission and assistance to perform the healing.

Mother Sarita carefully and respectfully and reverently passed the raw egg over Tim's body, beginning at his crown and going down the left shoulder and down and up the left arm, down and up the left leg, down and up the right leg, up to the right shoulder and down and up the right arm back to the crown of his head. She then held the egg for another prayer. Then into the glass of water set on the altar at the beginning, she cracked the egg putting the shells in a small frying pan and putting them aside. She held the glass up for each of us to see and explained what was being shown. There were distinct patterns that the yolk and white formed following the shape of a body with knots in them, showing the problems in Tim's body, and the water was murky. Mother Sarita explained to Tim that his spiritual receptors were blocked and his body was unable to process the information it needed to be well. What I didn't know at that time was Tim had HIV AIDS. With several more prayers, she poured the water and egg into the frying pan with the shells and frankincense, myrrh and copal wood. We all then proceeded outside to a fire that was hot and ready into which she deposited the concoction with more passionate prayers asking that this condition be corrected. That was the end of session one. I had a million questions and the configurations of the egg in the water were undeniable.

At that moment, Mother Sarita's son Miguel came in to say hello. He had copies of his book, *The Four Agreements*, and gave us each a copy, which I gladly accepted. When I read it, I thought he wrote it just for me. Books like that always found me one way or the other.

It was week two and we all gathered again. This time, Anne Marie, the new volunteer subject, wanted to know if she was pregnant and if the pregnancy was viable. We repeated the prescribed prayers and ceremonial process, and as Mother Sarita held up the glass, we were in awe. The egg white showed the shape of a fetus and the umbilical cord perfectly attached to the yoke. The water was clear and the egg white was luminescent. The prognosis was a viable healthy pregnancy. We finished the spiritual inquiry, and I was speechless as the realization of our interrelated universe crept into my experiential awareness.

Weeks three and four, we each had the privilege of passing the egg over the volunteer subject's body, cracking it into the water and diagnosing the results under the direction of Mother Sarita. I was very at home with this process given my intuition and interpretation of the spirit world experiences. I didn't know exactly what we all had just experienced in terms of the over-all picture of spiritual energy healing, but I did feel like I had found home, and the matrix of learning that was my spiritual healing life began to come together with greater meaning and serendipity.

What I was beginning to realize was that, because of the global and galactic organic nature of the multitude of energy healing practices, it was difficult if not impossible to understand. It came to me that one way I could help was to create a "yellow pages" to assist others to find and learn about this field. That was before the Internet!

What I am sharing here from my life experience and research is the broad categorical description of the many kinds of energy healing referred to as the new medicine for the new human in this new world. The exciting part about this is this can be a foundation for Internet research around anything that draws your interest. I do this with the hope and intent that it will accelerate the awareness and understanding of this ancient/new indispensable body of healing opportunities, and consequently contribute to your high level of health, well-being and spiritual evolution being demanded by the times.

Holistic Energy Healing Modalities - Descriptive Categories and Names

Holistic Energy Healing is a process of discovering, diagnosing, correcting and/or promoting the correct flow of energy in accordance with the correct electromagnetic energy, light and information and universal laws. This is done with the intent of recovering the dynamic balance that allows optimum health and well-being.

This healing and balancing is often body-centered, however, that includes the total individual field of energy and the universal field that is all-inclusive of all living things. The description of the field will be presented in detail in the next section.

Some of the modalities are not identified as holistic energy healing methods, but do affect the flow of energy because everything is energy and everything is connected...part of the whole. This applies to all things in creation, physical and non-physical, multidimensional configurations and entities, physical spaces and social, political, or religious configurations. Remember that nothing is separate, so there is overlap of technique, intent and purpose in these categories. It is important to be aware that all methods and therapies involve the energy system, physical, mental, emotional and spiritual and environmental aspects of life. This information defies strict categorization or total inclusion of all healing methods in many ways, and is for the purpose of functional, foundational knowledge to assist you on your healing journey.

Eleven Categories of Over 180 Holistic Energy Healing Methods

1. Healing Performed By A Practitioner Using Hands On Or Hands In The Field Techniques:

Cranial Sacral Work, Reiki, Massage, Healing Touch, Acupressure, Reflexology, Lymph Drainage, Laying on of Hands, Deeksha, Blessings, Psychic Surgery, NLP, Therapeutic Touch, Pranic Healing, Rolfing, Abayanga, Still Point, Matrix Energetics, Reconnection Healing

2. Healing Performed By A Practitioner Using Hands, Manipulation And/Or Instruments On Or Near The Body:

Acupuncture, Chiropractic, Osteopathy, Surgery, Physical Therapy, Nursing, Kinesthesiology, Magnetic Therapies

3. Healing Performed Using Machines And/Or Instruments On Or Near The Body:

Dowsing, Pendulum Measurements, Tesla Lights, Laser and Light Therapy, Computerized Vibrational Detection Reading Methods, Bio-feedback

4. Healing Created Through Inspiration And Spiritual Practices:

Prayer, Clergy, Speakers, Music, Theater, Books, Nature, Actions, Experiences, Philosophy, Affirmations, Religious Ceremony, Practices and Beliefs, Cultural Morays, History, Counseling, Coaching

5. Healing Created Through Body-Centered Participatory Physical Methods:

Dance, Yoga, Tai Chi, Chi Gung, Tapping, Energy Medicine, Kundalini Yoga, Feldenkrais, Heller Work, Nia, Zumba, Ropes, Heart Math, Pranayama, Chanting, Sweat Lodges, Moving Meditation, Free Dance, Creative Dance, Trance Dance, Buzz Method, Melt Technique, Egoscue Method, Challenging Activities such as Cross-Fit, Ropes, Personal Quests, Individual Sports such as Triathlons, Marathons, etc.

6. Healing Created Through Body-Centered And Mental Methods:

Hypnosis, Biofeedback, Brain Gym, Mind Math, EMDR, TheWork, Experiential Education, Creative Visualization, Guided Visualization

7. Healing Created With Sound, Rhythm And Vibration To Entrain And Balance The Field:

Gong, Drums, Crystal Bowls, Tibetan Bowls, Specific Music, Chanting, Mantra, Electronic Tones

8. Healing Created Through Body-Centered, Meridian-Based, And/Or Psychological Methods:

Talk Therapy, Psychotherapy, Cognitive Therapy, Behavioral Therapy, Energy Psychology, EFT, TFT, TAT, CEP, and numerous others, Emotional Fitness, Soul Detective Work, Energy Medicine, Body Talk, Chakra Healing, Kundlini Yoga, Shadow Work, Dream Work, Earthing and Journaling

9. Healing Created With Guided Activities To Create Altered States Of Consciousness:

Meditation, Hynotherapy, Quantum Jumping, Trance Dance, Drumming, Ceremony, Ritual, Prayer, Resonant Healing, White, Red and Black Tantric, Pranayam, Ethnic Dance

10. Healing Created By Using Natural And/Or Synthetic Substances To Create Altered States Of Health, Healing And/Or Awareness:

Naturopathy, Homeopathy, Aromatherapy, Ayahauska Ceremony, Peyote Ceremony, Pharmaceutical Substances, Specific Foods, Supplements and Herbs, Ayurvedic Remedies, San Pedro, Ibogaine Treatment, Psilocybin Mushrooms

11. Healing In The Multidimensional Spiritual Realm:

Past Life Healing, Soul Retrieval, Medium Reading, Spiritual Intuition, Soul Detective Work, Transpersonal Healing, Surrogate Healing, Channeling, Shamanism, Emotional Fitness, Clairvoyant, Clairaudient, Remote Viewing and Remote Healing, Soul Retrieval, Matrix Re-patterning, Native American Animal Medicine, Shape Shifting, Resonant Healing, Clairsentient, Psychokinetic, Psychic Reading, Exorcism, Training in Power Methods, Clairsniffient

Summary of the Galactic View of Holistic Energy Healing Possibilities

We are so fortunate to live in these times of unlimited opportunity for optimum health and well-being and understanding of our true identity. We are supported by ancient healing traditions, amazing leading edge scientific discoveries about our body, mind and spirit healing capabilities. We have unprecedented access to the knowledge, awareness and experience of the needs of our bodies, hearts and souls and deepest desires, for ourselves, our loved ones, our personal, global and galactic societies and environments.

My declared and realized soul's purpose has been to be a catalyst for evolutionary healing and self-realization universal principles and methods. I am grateful for my very fortunate and fulfilling life. Writing this book is a dream come true and I thank you as a reader. It is my deepest desire that this information serves you in realizing your dreams in a way that would be otherwise not possible.

So You Want to Know Your Life's Purpose?!

The purpose of life is a life of purpose.

-Robert Byrne

One of the most common questions I hear is, "What is my life's purpose?" What I know for sure is our souls know why we are here. Our families, societies, religions, schools and professions most often dictate purpose and offer models and images or possibilities of purpose. The problem is in these cases, we are largely described and defined with words, concepts, roles and personalities, all of which apply in our socioeconomic circles, but is often a language our souls don't speak. To add to the difficulty of knowing your life's purpose, historically, the importance of purpose has been defined through competition, outward signs of success, approval, brilliance, extent of impact on the world, notoriety and fame, and are largely external descriptions and transient at best.

The Master Keys to Unlocking Who You Really Are - Self-Image and Self-Identity

Know thyself.

- Socrates

I was seven and it was summer vacation. I had dressed in my cotton shorts and triangle top that tied in front which my Mom had sewn for me. It was freshly pressed and I liked the lavender and white floral pattern the most, and the way it went with my white shorts and tennies. Mom had braided my hair and I had done my chores and then stole away with my dog, Molly, to my favorite playground...the foothills above our house. I had no thought of what my life purpose was, I was clearly doing what I spontaneously felt was the most important thing and I wanted to be unencumbered by "shoulds."

I passed all the familiar and reassuring natural landmarks and some I had made to find my way back. And I remembered that Hansel and Gretel had not been wise leaving bread crumbs, although I had brought some crackers for the ants and the birds and a small bottle of water for me and Molly. I liked to go where I could no longer see any houses and I felt like a true adventurer about to make more incredible discoveries (I really haven't changed much since then). I began slowing down and looking carefully at the rocks where I could easily find small fossils, for this land used to be a lake. My imaginary friends would gather, and Molly seemed to know them and we would play. Birds would come for the crackers and I would always crumble one on the anthill and watch the ants say thank you as they hauled the crumbs into their hill home. We would play guessing games, imagining games, make fun shadows, or pretend it was still a lake, find-the-best-fossil and prettiest-plant-games. I would feel like a Native Indian and time would disappear. Life was good and I had no questions. When I got hungry, I knew it was time to go back home.

It was many years later after a childhood of seeking approval, achievement, trying and succeeding in fitting in, high school, college, marrying and having children and returning to school, did the question of my life's purpose come up for me. What I first realized was that my life had become about other people's approval and expectations, societal norms and my own conditioned unconscious beliefs that had been running my recent, not so purposeful, life.

It was a good life, one many would have loved to live and I enjoyed it, but the sense that something was missing drove me to introspection (a childhood coping mechanism) and an even more intense study of other cultures, cultural anthropology, and again, asking why people do the things they do. I actually considered being a roving reporter at one time. I began many spiritual pursuits and began training in Astrology (to prove it was not valid), Pranayam (the use of the breath for healing), Native American, South American and Chinese Healing Sciences. What I didn't know, was this was the beginning of my understanding of my life's purpose, for it was the beginning of my remembering my true essence and identity at a spiritual level in terms of feeling and inner-knowing. This was a level which was for the most part silent, and I could dip into a feeling of wholeness and familiarity which reminded me of the natural self-acceptance I experienced as a child.

I have found that those who ask what their life purpose is almost always also say they want to recapture an earlier time in their lives when they were happier, freer and felt better about themselves. After many years of research, consulting, counseling and facilitating holistic and energy healing, this is what I have come to believe about life purpose.

Everyone's life purpose is the same... **Manifest from consciousness/ pure potentially that which is your deepest driving desire for life using your unique gifts and abilities in service to others.**

The initial problem with this statement is it is lovely and inspirational, but practically meaningless without the following considerations:

- You cannot know your true life's purpose and be happy if you do not know yourself at the level of your Soul.
- You cannot know your life's purpose and be happy if you do not realize and have gratitude for your unique personage and gifts.
- You cannot know your life's purpose and be happy if you do not live a life of service to others.
- You cannot know your life's purpose and be happy without living it.

So the question is not what is my life's purpose? It is really four questions:

1. Do I know and experience myself at the level of my Soul?
2. Am I willing to be open to, know the value of, understand and be grateful for my unique gifts and talents?
3. Am I present for whatever life offers and do I live in the awareness of serving others using my unique gifts as my life purpose?
4. Am I willing to co-create my life story as a positive legacy with each thought, word and action in fulfillment of my life purpose?

It is my intention to assist you in being able to answer "Yes!" to each of the questions above, for then you will not only know your life purpose, but you will be living it as only you can. And so, we will set about discovering the very exciting answers to the seemingly mundane questions below:

NowOpp@WhoAreYou?

Just a current reality check: Briefly answer these questions here and now for future reference:

- Who are you?
- Where do you live?
- Why are you here?
- What laws do you live by?
- What keys are on your key ring?
- What languages do you speak?
- Who is on your life consulting team?

Section Three

The Real Truth of Who You Really Are

Learning To Be Who You Are Not

Before I was five years old, I unconsciously figured out through "behavioral trial and error" that if I didn't like the way things were going I could change the situation by getting angry.

If no one would listen to me or if I was being blamed for something I didn't do or being told something I didn't like, all I had to do was get angry, stomp upstairs to my room and slam the door. It worked, I was in the quiet and comfort of my room with all my favorite things and everyone left me alone and it was over.

After a while, I became aware that not everyone did this. In my family, my Mom would just stand her ground, my sister would disappear and my brother would patronize and lecture, usually me, and then leave for a more important activity. My friends had different ways of changing a situation too. Wendy would get real quiet and fake respectful, and then be real angry after; Joanne would get perfectly sweet and nice and cooperative; Ryan would go crazy, yell and scream and get in a lot of trouble and get grounded; Sylvia just did whatever she was told and never said a word or even showed an emotion; Donita didn't seem to want to change anything even if she didn't like it and it seemed like she was always sick anyway; Ethan would always blame someone or something else for whatever he didn't like; Kathy would just be perfect, get perfect grades, be the perfect student, daughter and church member and nothing ever bothered her; and the Andersons' strategy really caught my attention. It was unusual compared to the others. They would ask God for the right answer to absolutely every question. At their daily prayer meeting, all issues were addressed and resolved in some way. This was closer to the families depicted on television in those days. At this time, I didn't know I was witnessing the coping mechanisms and control strategies I would see throughout my life.

I grew to know my family and my friends' families and neighbors, in a way, through our defense, control or coping strategies. I wasn't conscious of that at the time, but looking back, I can remember knowing what would happen in any given situation at my house and each of my friend's houses or in the neighborhood. The way I interpreted it then was each household had certain spoken and/or unspoken rules about what you did when you were upset (or really excited) and when you were there, you followed their rules. This way

I learned to "communicate" and "fit in." And, of course, I wondered why each family had different rules and how they decided on them. The line of authority was never clear to me then.

What I understand now is I was assigning my own interpretation and practical definition and description to what I witnessed to figure out how to get along and try to make sense of it all and develop my own coping skills. What I was experiencing were energy dynamics of defense and/or control coping strategies. Although I felt something was missing, I didn't have an awareness of what wasn't being said or the emotions operating behind the dynamics, including my own at that age ...until I entered kindergarten.

I guess my Mom made me feel like everything was all right and I was all right, and the question that I wasn't, never came up. I believed in myself. My kindergarten teacher, Miss Finster, didn't. For her, everything was conditional and depended on how everyone behaved. That would have been ok, but how she interpreted how you behaved depended on whether she was having a good day or not. Also, if you had any needs outside of napping, milk time, play time and recess, or if the times scheduled for those activities didn't work for you, that was a problem. Feeling or expressing emotion was quickly reprimanded with no concern for why.

This was a whole new level of learning for me, and this was when I began to develop ways to manipulate my reality. Anger didn't work here and when I got a NS (not satisfactory) under "works and plays well with others" on my very first report card...I couldn't bear to be "Unsatisfactory" and I began to develop some new talents...fear-based thinking...acting like I didn't care and being "so perfect" that Miss Finster couldn't downgrade me. She won...and I lost some of my treasured spontaneity....but I didn't get any more NS's, and I had learned some new coping skills which served me well throughout my school years. The only problem was, by the time I entered college, I had lost an important part of myself and I really didn't know who I was, not an uncommon feeling for incoming college students.

Why am I telling you this story? Because we all have one...this was just mine, and quite gentle compared to so many seemingly insignificant childhood incidents that begin a domino effect of closing of doors to self-understanding, self-image, knowing what is correct and incorrect interaction, spontaneity, and authentic expression.

What I call the *OldKnew* medicine is really a way of undoing this and returning to the truth and experience of our true identity.

Becoming Who You Are

What I didn't learn in school has turned out to be the most important information of all. The blatantly absent knowledge and experience or a holistic approach from my school years has been shown to me in many fortunate ways...through my strong and very spiritual Mother, through my beloved pets, through all forms of nature, through teachers and clergy who knew how to teach to think in terms of possibilities, and through dreams, sensations, ideas, thoughts and desires of unknown origin to me, which I now know as the grace of God. These were the treasured keys that opened the doors to the understanding of my life's purpose as a seeker, intuitive, researcher, integrator, writer, author and teacher.

We are all given these clues and keys in some way, and the purpose of this book is to be one of those ways for whoever chooses to read it. In terms of information, knowledge and experience of the spiritual expansion of heightened conscious awareness, the merging agreement about the nature of life between scientists and sages is accelerating the return to the truth of who we are.

If there were a few little known facts, a few tested techniques and just a few shifts in your perception that could make a difference for you between a mediocre or compromised life and a magnificent life, would you be interested? If a fear-based life could become a confidence-based life rid of emotional turmoil and disappointment and filled with peace, love and harmony, would you like to know how? You might find this a lofty promise and your life experience may have shown you this is not likely, but I encourage you to read on because this is not just an inspirational, self-help book. It is energetically powerful.

Light Through the Key Hole is an account of the little known facts (secrets) about our true identity prescribed by ancient knowledge, made evident by current awareness and validated by leading edge scientific findings. I call this the OldKnew knowledge...unknown and/or unavailable before that has been the key keepers of our reality. These OldKnew technologies now available to all provide the learning experience necessary to unlock the doors that have been the obstacles to our knowing and living our authentic selves. Through making just a few shifts you will be led to your permanent and sustainable transformation. In fact, it is a transmutation of your conscious awareness and consequent experience of your own joy, reliable knowing, excellence, and magnificence...your true identity... as your way of life. This finally answers the age old question correctly for you from the inside out about who you are, and why you are here.

Who in the World Do You Think You Are?

Your true identity is known by a felt sense and inner-knowing rather than an intellectual sense or outer-knowing and is most likely beyond your current comprehension in terms of all of who you really are. It takes knowledge, awareness and experience to truly know yourself, but we cannot think ourselves to the realization of our true identity. A complete and successful pursuit of true identity and purpose must come from a complete approach of study, expanded awareness, and spiritual practice. We then open to the truth of who we are and it is realized and experienced from within. You may wonder why I am so sure of this...

Well, I never really believed much in visions. At the very least I thought they were just for very holy people or sages or seers, or someone with mental problems. It was a time in my life when I was meditating regularly, doing a lot of hiking, deep in study of philosophy, religion and multicultural healing, which was part of my pursuit for meaning and breakthroughs. I felt quite balanced, but stuck, in a way, between my now mainstream life and my deep driving desire to be "out in the field of all possibilities." I couldn't seem to integrate those two aspects of my life.

It was late, about 10:30 P.M., and I was tired, but I had a workshop beginning the next day and wanted to look my best. I decided to put a cleansing clay mask on my face. It was to be left on only seven minutes and then I could wash my face and go to sleep. I made the mask and put it on and had the thought to lie down for the seven minutes. I fell sound asleep quickly.

Suddenly, I was aware of nothing less than the Mother-Father God standing at the foot of my bed. I still don't know if I had my eyes open or closed, but they were incredibly beautiful standing in loving surrounding iridescent light together as one the Father on my right and the Mother on my left dressed in white and pale blue robes. The Mother wore what appeared to be a rosary with beads and crystals as a necklace and the Father had beads in his left hand. And then they spoke kindly with one, to voice:

"The space between your thoughts and your feelings is Lucifer's playground."

I could feel my heart expand, but suddenly my awareness went to my face which felt like it was on fire. The clay had dried and I don't know how long I had been asleep. I leapt out of bed and went into the bathroom to wash the clay off. I splashed some cool water on my face and the clay began to wash away. As I looked in the mirror again, the Mother and Father were now standing behind me, the Father on my right and the Mother on my left, and now I was standing in the golden loving light with them. They spoke once more: "Your thoughts cloud the truth of who you really are. Just feel and you can know the truth."

This time, I didn't move in a semi-conscious attempt to savor this incredible experience, but the light dissipated and my attention went back to the burning sensation on my face.

I finished washing my face and it was beet red and still stinging. I put some calming lotion on and just stood there for a few minutes trying to understand what just happened. I went back to bed trying to bring some normalcy back and don't really remember lying down or falling asleep, but woke up refreshed and renewed and with a heartfelt sense of peace and understanding.

That marked a turning point in my life and in my work...opening to the "unknown," less thinking and more feeling to learn, know and understand.

The Anatomy of Your Soul - The Whole Truth about You

The kingdom of God is within you and all around you.

-Gospel of Thomas

The preschool and early elementary school experience was quite the education for me, indeed.

I had some vague idea that I was not just a physical body, a mind and personality, although traditional curriculums did not support that idea. Physical education or health education was more about what we didn't talk about as what we did talk about. The subjects of sex and menstruation were handled by a small brochure handed out discretely. There was no discussion about any "unseen aspects" of our physicality or health. In fact the word "unseen" used with physical was a conundrum. And knowledge of anatomy was at a bare, bare minimum. All subjects were taught separately as if they had nothing to do with each other.

I had no concept of actually being a soul, spirit. In my religious, church and spiritual education, I learned my spirit was outside of me in heaven, wherever that was...and I was called an angel from time to time, which didn't really resonate because they were in heaven too. I never thought about how I knew things that hadn't happened yet or were things not in sight, smell, taste or touch...They just materialized in my mind and I didn't question it.

A lot of the time I felt that I was my thoughts, opinions and behaviors. I formed my self-image largely by my experiences, with the exception of my dear Mother's encouraging words and discouraging words from teachers sometimes. I learned very quickly in elementary school that no one wanted to hear things that were unknowable. I also noticed that none of the other kids knew unknown stuff or at least they weren't saying so.

And so, through the tender young ages of six through ten, I learned to be quiet and feel somehow wrong, and when unexpected things would happen, or I would discover that I was out of the regularly accepted normal, my very identity was shaken. It wasn't all that bad to just do what I was told, but it did feel a bit fake and hollow to me. And the primer readers were exceptionally boring and unimaginative to me. And so I went about developing skills to fit in and get along and get recognized for being a bright, well-behaved young girl.

From that point on, I was destined to go "main stream" and see how much I could achieve. I lived largely in the real world but with what I like to call an unrequited truth seeking syndrome that I satisfied by spending a lot of time alone with my dog and in nature with all my largely reliable spirit friends. That worked quite well and no one really noticed.

It took me all the way to my sophomore year in college to run across a class that made mention of something other than the physical, psychological, or emotional aspects of our being. While fulfilling my undergraduate requirements, I luckily chose Advanced Physical Education and ended up with a professor who made yoga mandatory once a week. That singular elective class was the turning point back to the knowing the "unknown" internal world. I couldn't wait for the class each week and during Savasana (relaxation at the end of class) I would drift off into that joyous, judgeless, pure potential place I had longed for. That yoga class along with Philosophy and Psychology started opening the doors to access the missing pieces (unanswered questions) with which I had been grappling.

After many years, I eventually came to know what I knew in the first place at some deep innocent level, that we are far more than a physical body, mind and personality, titles, roles, careers or accomplishments. We are spiritual beings, primarily spiritual and etheric in nature, and a detection and communication system second to none. We are the unknown and the unknowable. We meet ourselves through experience. Holistic studies and spiritual practices create that experience of our true identity.

Anatomy 202 Or What Your Anatomy Teacher (If You Had One) Didn't Know Or Didn't Tell You

Who do you think you are? What do you think of yourself? What is your self-image? Why is this so important? Because your entire experience of life depends first on what is your perception of yourself. It determines your interpretation of all that is, all that you experience and all that you desire. If you do not know the core of your existence and identity, your truth cannot be known.

You are phenomenal beyond your current comprehension. You are so magnificent that you must incorporate your imagination and your ability to feel to even begin to comprehend. You are a complete and complex luminous energy field matrix capable of anything you can imagine, unique, irreplaceable, and with unlimited comprehension and ability. You are not simply a body, mind and spirit. Close your eyes (unless you are driving) right now and felt sense the truth of that.

It is very important for your correct self-knowledge and self-image, and to begin to realize your limitless personal power and have an experiential understanding of your unbounded, divine identity and true spiritual nature and your life's real purpose. This knowledge is also important for the foundation to understand how the OldKnew technologies work to heal imbalances, for this is the field that encompasses all the systems you are, seen and unseen. This is where and how healing and transformation take place and the proper flow of prana is reestablished. In addition, with the awareness of this true identity, we can come to understand the interrelatedness of the universe, our unique place in the universe and our unique purpose. Your unseen energy system is learned through felt sense and sensation and expanded awareness.

NowOpp@MyEnergyMatrix

Simply put your attention on the image on the next page and then close your eyes. Take a deep breath and turn your awareness inward and allow your field to have your attention through sensation and imagination. Go on an adventure and find the chakras, meridians and your biofield, and as that witness, just allow it to come into your awareness in any way it does. This also serves as a NowOpp@Nonjudgment. Your experience will just be as it is and that will be perfect. There is no right or wrong way to do this meditation...except to be judgemental about it.

The Human Biofield Matrix...You...Inside Out and Outside In.

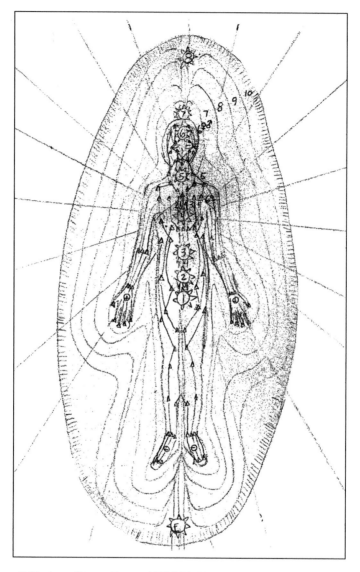

8 Chakras (Power Centers) 72,000 Meridians (Energy Channels)
10 Bodies (Spectrums of Vibration) 50 to 75 Trillion Magnificent Cells
A microcosm of the macrocosm and inextricably connected to all things through Prana

Meet Your Ten Bodies

If you understand that you are Ten Bodies, and you are aware of those Ten Bodies, and you keep them in balance; the whole universe will be in balance within you.

- Yogi Bhajan, Ph.D.

You have ten bodies or ranges of vibratory existence. One of them is your physical body. Three are mental bodies and six are etheric bodies. They make up your field of energy. All of them have powerful special capacities and special gifts. Again, simply contemplate the potentiality of this knowledge to further your understanding of yourself beyond the finite and beyond right and wrong.

1. Soul Body - connects you to your inner infinity. It is the experience of the flow of spirit within you. When it is strong, you live from your heart and your life flows with ease. If it is weak, you may feel stuck and unable to access your purpose and creative flow.
2. Negative or Protective Mind – If it is well-developed, gives you the gifts of containment, form and discernment. It gives you patience to be obedient to your higher inner-guidance. If it is underdeveloped, your longings can cause you to get into inappropriate, self-destructive relationships and be over-influenced by others because you are not contained enough in your own center.
3. Positive or Expansive Mind – sees the positive essence of all situations and beings. It is expansive and allows resources in. It gives you a strong will and allows you to use your power easily and humbly. It makes you naturally playful and optimistic and gives you a good sense of humor. If it is weak, it is like poison. You can be overwhelmed by the input of your Negative Mind which can be depressing and paralyzing. You may be angry or intolerant or hesitant because of too much fear.
4. Neutral or Meditative Mind – is the ultimate "win-win" mentality. Being established in a neutral or meditative state allows you to look at all of life with compassion, including yourself. The neutral/meditative mind evaluates the input of your Negative and Positive Mind and all the bodies, and gives you guidance within nine seconds. It gives you an intuitive vantage point and allows you to

access your Soul. If it is weak, you still have trouble with making decisions. You'll have the habit of feeling victimized and will be unable to integrate your experiences and find meaning in them.

5. <u>Physical Body</u> - is the temple where the other Nine Bodies play out their parts. It gives you the ability to balance all parts of your life. If strong, it is the teacher and brings information into concrete form. If it is weak, you may be angry, greedy, jealous, competitive, or ungrateful. Your inner and outer realities will be out of balance. You may have trouble expressing yourself.

6. <u>Arcline</u> – extends from earlobe to earlobe across the hairline and brow. It is your halo and the nucleus of the aura. Women have a second Arcline which extends from nipple to nipple. The Arcline is your projection, your radiance. It gives you the ability to focus, to concentrate and meditate. It is associated with the pituitary gland, regulates the nervous system and glandular balance. It is the balance point between the physical realm and the cosmic realm. If it is weak, you will be overprotective and easily influenced. You may have glandular imbalances, inconsistent moods and behavior. You may also not be using your intuition to protect yourself.

7. <u>Aura</u> – is the electromagnetic field which surrounds your body in the same way the Earth's Magnetic Field envelopes the Earth. When it is strong, it acts as a container for your life force and allows it to build, and your presence uplifts all. It will protect you from others' negativity. If it is weak, you may be paranoid and lack self-trust, suffer from negativity from other people or your psyche. Illness can result from this.

8. <u>Pranic Body</u> – continuously brings the life force into your system through your breath. This allows you to feel fearless and fully alive. All disease starts with an imbalance in the Pranic Body. If it is weak, you may have constant low-level anxiety and fatigue. You will have low energy and may be fearful and defensive.

9. <u>Subtle Body</u> – helps you see beyond the immediate realities of life to the subtle universal realities. When it is strong, you have greater finesse and a powerful calmness. You learn quickly and master situations easily. If it is weak, you may be naïve and easily fooled, unintentionally crude or rough in your speech or behavior. You may be restless, because you lack the peace that comes from a strong flowing subtle body.

10. <u>Radiant Body</u> – gives you spiritual royalty and radiance. When strong, it gives you courage in the face of any obstacle. You exert a magnetic presence and command respect of all who know you. If it is underdeveloped, you may be afraid of conflict. You may shy away from other people's attention, because you are afraid of the energy and responsibility that come with the recognition of your inner-nobility. You may feel ineffective and unable to come through in situations.

Where are You on the Metaphysical Map of Transformation?

Remember that we are timeless, multi-dimensional, energy beings. Intentional expansion of our conscious awareness will give us the experience and understanding at a cellular level of our true nature. In that state, our will is freed and we naturally allow ourselves to give up who we are not, to be who we are. This is the ultimate surrender. Sustainable transformation occurs at the vibrational level.

NowOpp@SpiritualBeingness

Please contemplate the map below and determine where your path has led or is leading you. This can serve as a point of reference for what you have manifested and possible revised direction and destination to the complete experience of your true destiny of spiritual beingness.

Energy Intent and Purpose	Quantum BioField Bodies	Energy Intent and Purpose
Fanatic in the Finite	Unbounded Oneness	Infinite
Loves Beliefs	Radiant	Loves Life
Wills Beliefs	Subtle	Divine Will same as Own Will
Fearful	Pranic	Trusting
Desires for Self Alone	Aura	Desires for Humanity
Overprotective and Paranoid	Arcline	Just and Humane
Exists for Validation	Physical	Balanced in Beingness
Thinks According to Beliefs	Neutral Mind	Discerning
Denial	Positive Mind	Potential
Blame	Negative Mind	Obedience to Universal Laws
Superior or Inferior Belief	Soul	Divine Being
Spiritual Unbeingness	Level of Vibration	Spiritual Beingness

Your Energy Channels and Treatment Points

Meridians are the Energy Channels that allow the life force to flow through you. Acupoints (there are upwards of 2,000 considered in Chinese Medicine/Acupuncture) on your skin along your meridians, are Activation Points for the stimulation of Pranic flow through your field used to correct, clear and balance the flow of the Life Force Energy throughout your field. In Energy Healing, we use just a few on 12 major meridians and two vessels. Not knowing about these is a little like not knowing you have blood vessels. This is key knowledge for the healing practices available to you.

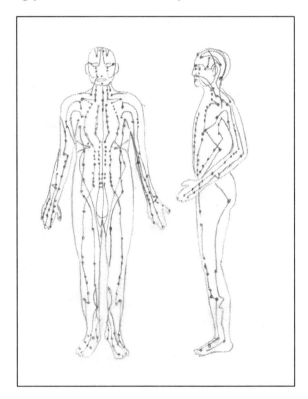

These drawings are meant to convey an idea of the fourteen major meridians (energy channels). There are 72,000 related meridians/channels and 2,000 + acupoints (energy healing treatment points). Due to space and angle limitations, all treatment points are not shown. These meridians and acupoints will be identified and explained in more detail later in the book.

The Eight Chakra Power Centers of Your Energy System

Below are the medical, physical and emotional aspects of each of the amazing Chakras (power centers) of the energy system. They are constantly taking in, synthesizing and integrating energy and information, and intricately interrelated to all other systems of the body and consequently instrumental in all types, clearing, balancing, healing and evolution. Not knowing about the chakras is a little like not knowing you have a heart.

NowOpp@MyChakras

Begin to familiarize yourself with the aspects of your chakras, the power centers of your Biofield. It will be helpful in your seeking and achieving and sustaining optimum health and well-being on all levels.

	First	Second	Third	Fourth	Fifth	Sixth	Seventh	Eighth
Location	Base of spine	Midway pubic bone to navel	Midway sternum to navel	Center of the chest	Throat	Center of forehead	Crown of head	Above the crown
Color	Red	Orange	Yellow	Green	Blue	Indigo	Violet	Gold White
Areas of Being	Stability, Security	Sensuality, creativity	Personal power and self-esteem	Love, harmony, nurturing	Communication and self-expression	Inspiration, intuition, insight	Connection and spirituality	Divinity, bliss
Glands	Endocrine	Reproductive	Adrenal	Thymus	Thyroid	Pituitary	Pineal	All
Organs and Body Parts	Large intestine, rectum, hips, and thighs	Organs of reproductive system, kidneys, and bladder	Liver, gallbladder, pancreas, spleen, small intestine, stomach	Heart, lungs, breasts	Throat, trachea, vocal chords	Eyes, ears, sinuses	Brain, hypothalamus	All biofield chakra meridians

			Personal power, moti-vated, decisive, willful, good self-image			Physic, visionary, imagina-tive, intuitive, percep-tive	Universal con-scious-ness, uncon-ditional love, enlight-enment, higher aware-ness	Oneness, whole-ness, beyond thought, self-help, timeless, space-less
When Open and In Balance	Cen-tered, safety, secure, grounded	Patient, endur-ing, self-con-fident, well-being		Accept-ance, love, fulfilled, harmony	Expres-sive, creative, commu-nicative			
When Closed or Out of Balance	Self-indul-gence, self-centere-dness, inse-curity, instabil-ity, grief, depres-sion	Frustra-tion, anxiety, fear, frig-idness, over-whelmed	Power-less, greedy, low self-esteem, doubt, anger, guilt, ag-gression	Loneli-ness, insen-sitivity, extreme emo-tions, closed, passive, sadness, overly selfless	Stagna-tion, sup-pressed, obses-sion, lack of expres-sion, lack of commu-nication, untruth	Difficulty focusing, detach-ment, intellec-tual stag-nation, fuzzy thinking	Con-fined, alone-ness, skepti-cal, accusa-tional, hateful	Desper-ate, hopeless, isolated, lost, frag-mented, superior or infe-rior
Health Effects When Closed or Out of Balance	Hemor-rhoids, consti-pation, sciatica	Infertil-ity, PMS, meno-pause difficulty, kidney/bladder problems	Diabetes, ulcers, poor di-gestion, jaundice, hepa-titis, hypo-gly-cemia, gall-stones	Breast/lung, heart, and immune diseases; high blood pressure, stroke, arthritis	Sore throat, laryngi-tis, stut-tering, thyroid problems	Eye diseases, hearing loss, schizo-phrenia, head-aches	Depres-sion, psy-chosis, epilepsy, brain tumors, cranial pressure	Insanity, suicidal, chronic depres-sion, anxiety, despair, delusion

The energetic, spiritual aspects of the Chakras used for meditation and energy balancing showing the frequencies that balance and tone the system when toned and spinning correctly

Location	Quality	Color	Aroma	Mantra	Key
Base of Spine	Stability	Red	Cedar	Lam	C
Abdomen	Sexuality	Orange	Gardenia	Vam	D
Solar Plexus	Desire	Yellow	Carnation	Ram	E
Heart	Peace	Green	Jasmine	Yum	F
Throat	Communication	Blue	Frankincense	Hum	G
Third Eye	Insight	Indigo	Sandalwood	Kshum	B
Crown	Enlightenment	Violet	Lotus	Ohm	A
18" above Crown	Bliss	Opalescence White	Rose	Silence	All Sound

NowOpp@ChakraMeditation

While seated comfortably, using the energetic and spiritual aspects of the Chakras chart above, put your attention on each chakra at the location indicated. Consider the quality of that chakra and breath in a deep breath of the color of the chakra into the chakra, then imagine the aroma and say or think the mantra (healing sound) for that chakra. When you have completed all eight chakras, take a deep breath, close your eyes and allow your chakra energy to integrate. When ready and rested, open your eyes.

More Amazing Belief-Gap-Producing Revelations You Need To Know

Everyone wants to be right, but no one stops to consider if their idea of right is right.

-F.M. Alexander

The Human body is made up of (depending on which scientist you ask) 60 to 90 trillion molecular geniuses – our cells. Thanks to the amazing scientific research community and technology, and the medical community, we know more about those cells and our body's functions than ever before in history, and there is a lot of good news. To add to our foundational knowledge is this very brief introductory look at four particular scientific findings and one diagnostic procedure that stand out as extremely evolutionary and particularly beneficial possibilities and compatibility in terms of scientific support for outcomes of holistic energy healing.

Neuroplaticity – Your Brain Isn't What You Thought It Was

Neuroscientists have determined the brain is not a static organ with pre-determined intelligence and function, but dynamic and has the capability to change structure and function, reorganize neural pathways and networks, and change their connections and behavior in response to new information, sensory stimulation and nutrition.

What this means is the brain functions can be determined by the way the brain is used, and the conscious healing use of the brain and care of the brain can change the brain.

Most of our body's cells die and are replaced every few weeks or months. Neurons, the primary cell of the nervous system do not multiply for the most part after we are born and are as old as we are. The cells are the same, but the connections change based on their/ our experience. A single nervous system has over 1 trillion cells. Our entire body is made up of 60 to 90 trillion cells that work together to generate perfect health. (Internet search - neuroplasticity)

Book Resource:
Super Brain, by Deepak Chopra, M.D. and R.E. Tanzi, Ph.D.

The String Theory AKA the Theory of Everything

The ancients intuited that time is eternal and everything in creation is connected by the same electromagnetic energy and light and that everything, manifest or unmanifest, is made of the same energy and vibration. The String Theory essential idea, is that all the different fundamental particles of the Standard Model of matter are really just different manifestations of one basic object: a string. Even though there is no direct experimental evidence that the developing String Theory is a correct description of Nature, we know that under an extremely powerful microscope that the string can oscillate in different ways and appear to be a photon, electron or a quark. So if this theory is correct, the entire world is made of strings! And that would agree with the ancient intuited knowledge that the whole universe is made of endless and interconnected light and energy. (www.superstringtheory.com)

The implications of scientists and sages coming together in agreement and validating and expanding the terms of our spiritual nature and connectedness with all things are extremely promising in eliminating pain and suffering. In addition, the reality that spiritually or scientifically we are all indeed connected, supports the fact that when we heal ourselves, through our connectedness, others heal as well. Adhering to the holistic healing premise that nothing is separate encourages clearing and creating the best environment for our trillions of helpers helping them efficiently complete the self-healing, co-creative miracle processes.

Our Bodies Are Our Subconscious Mind

The fabulous findings of Candace Pert, Ph.D., pharmacologist, research professor and author of *Molecules of Emotions*, demonstrate that every cell in the body is studded with hundreds of thousands of receptor molecules programmed to bind with peptides or information substances to guide our bodies responses to inner and outer cues. Thanks to Dr. Pert's work, we now understand that what Freud termed the subconscious mind is actually a measurable physical process and physiological underpinnings of the effects of thoughts and emotional events on our physical well-being, and shows the absolute interrelatedness of the body and mind.

In her spoken presentation of *Your Body is Your Subconscious*, Dr. Pert discusses how her findings are also beginning to reveal the underlying functions of the energy system and views of the chakras as "minibrains" that receive, process and distribute information from and to the rest of the body/mind or field. Also, that the neuronal functions reflect the spiritual attributes associated with the corresponding chakras.

It is theorized that every cell in the body has memory capability and that the cells in the gut actually have greater memory capability than the cells of the brain. There is not total agreement over the theory called, "Cellular Memory," however, circumstances of phantom pain from amputated limbs, and heart transplant patients having memories and personality traits of the donor, provide fuel to the debate and demonstrate a possible energetic memory blueprint.

When I met Candace, a delightful person, many years ago, she was a dyed-in-the-wool research-scientist, it-doesn't-exist-if-it-can't-be-proven-in-lab doctor. As a result of her research and understanding and experience of the human body, mind and spirit, she now speaks on Science and Spirituality, and authored, *The Scientific Basis Behind Mind-Body Medicine, Everything You Need to Know to Feel Go(o)d)*, and the Musical Chakra Guided Imagery CD, *Psychosomatic Wellness: Healing your Body-Mind*. (www.candacepert.com)

Hydrating – Seems Obvious, However...Dehydration is Devastating to All Efforts

Where is your water?

From the Hopi Elders Message

There is no disagreement that I know of, except perhaps in rare medical cases, that we need an adequate amount of water for optimum health and well-being. Every system in your body depends on water. For example, water flushes toxins out of vital organs, carries nutrients to your cells and provides a moist environment for ear, nose and throat tissues. Lack of water can lead to dehydration, a condition that occurs when you don't have enough water in your body to carry out normal functions. Even mild dehydration can drain your energy and make you tired.

We are made up mainly of water and electrical current. The electrical current cannot flow properly without adequate water, and neither can any of our body's systems work correctly. Weight loss and/or maintaining optimum weight is difficult if you are not adequately hydrated.

I know you have heard this before. Do you drink enough water? Enough said, make it a priority. Devise schemes, strategies and arrangements to make it happen. Although there is some disagreement about how much we need and when, here is what I find to be close to the most common recommendations from health organizations, professionals, trainers, and healers. Energy work, meditation, yoga and pretty much everything else does not go as well if you are not adequately hydrated.

1. Drink the purest water you can, as needed. (If that is reverse osmosis water, add a pinch of sea-salt to each gallon)
2. Eat high water content foods, fruits, fresh vegetables
3. Drink one half your body weight in ounces.
   (120 pounds = 60 ounces)
4. Drink 2 glasses first thing and/or 30 minutes before eating in the morning (2)
5. Drink 1 glass 30 minutes before each meal (3)

6. Drink 1 glass before going to bed (1)
   (Adjust the ounce size to your needs: 60 ounces = six 10-ounce glasses)
   Note: If you drink sodas, caffeinated tea, coffee, alcohol or other sweet or artificially sweetened drinks, drink the same ounces of water to compensate
   Note: Herbal tea can count as water
   Note: Adjust water amount up for extra exercise or exposure to high temperatures or dry climates

Resource Guide:
Your Body's Many Cries for Water, by Fereydoon Batmangheilid, M.D.

The Universal Energy Healing Heart Massage

This is a priceless, quick healing tool to heal, resolve obstacles we come up against, and sustain good pranic flow throughout our field for optimum health and well-being. It is based on the energetic anatomy we have just been introduced to and the premises of energy psychology.

What we've found out so far:

- We are light, energy and information
- Connected to all things
- Our bodies are our subconscious
- Our true nature is one of harmony, peace and purpose
- Prana, the life force, moves through our field and we have an energy system with chakras (power centers), meridians (channels) and a biofield (layers of energy) to receive and give pranic energy
- Anything other than harmony, peace and purpose is due to an interruption in the energy system
- We can correct incorrect pranic flow by stimulating flow through our energy system using the acupoints or the chakras while focusing mentally on certain issues. (Preview of Energy Psychology, which is addressed under the Extraordinary Section)

NowOpp@UniversalHealingHeartMassage

This healing technique goes as follows.

Take some deep Breaths and be sure you are hydrated.

Think of an emotion, thought or situation that is causing you pain or turmoil.

Rate it on a scale of 1 – 10 (1-2 is it is annoying, 9 -10 is it is debilitating). This is a subjective rating, and if you wish you can use muscle testing (see next page) to test which number is most accurate.

Now place the palm of one of your hands on the center of your chest, the heart chakra. Make a circle up towards the left shoulder and down and around up to the right shoulder back to where you started. (That is clockwise if the clock is on your chest)

As you are circling your hand, say "Even though I feel, or I am (anxious, depressed, angry, out of shape, confused, sad, etc.)_____, I completely accept and love myself. (c.a.l.m.) Repeat this three times. Keep saying how you feel with this statement taking deep breaths between sentences. Say it exactly how it is. Use the statements: "Even if I never get over this _____, I completely accept and love myself." And I respect my feelings and ideas and thoughts about this and I completely accept and love myself. Just two or three minutes should help. Sometimes other issues come up with the process, so just include them too.

Now take some deep breaths and be sure you are properly hydrated.

Rate the issue again and see where you are. Repeat the process if necessary.

What this does is release the interruption, so the energy can move and resolve. It enables you to be more neutral and calm about whatever the issue is.

If you wish, and it feels true to you, you can do the heart circle and say positive affirmations in acknowledgement relief from the issue that was bothering you.

For example, "Even though I felt really angry, I feel ok now." And repeat it three times.

You can try this on everything; it is harmless, empowering and helpful.

Muscle Testing - The Truth, the Whole Truth and Nothing but the Truth

What if we had a diagnostic technique that could objectively measure truth, truth beyond memory and the mind, truth that makes you free? Well, we do! And it is the diagnostic gift of muscle testing.

Our connectedness and interrelatedness with all things is supported by the phenomenal relatively new healing truth measuring tool of Muscle Testing, also called energy testing and energy checking.

Even though it appears we are testing the strength or weakness of muscles, what we are really testing is the free or obstructed and/ or interrupted flow of energy and the effect those states have on the physiology. It is simply a refinement that I believe helps understand the function and language of the body.

Never before in the history of humanity has a tool like this existed. It has been a game changer for many areas of application for diagnosis and for preventative health care such allergies, nutrition, psychiatry, stress, mental emotional fitness, self-knowledge, self-realization, and now is indispensable in holistic energy healing protocols, therapies and technologies.

Historically, facts or diagnosis and/or preventive steps have depended on opinion, professional observation and consulting various manuals of symptoms, beliefs, debates, dogmas, philosophies, mandates, scientific proof and recorded events. So much of what was considered to be true was representative of collective beliefs, theory, statistics, categorization, classification, odds, percentages and repeated experience, and not purely objective. This has shaped the face of today's health care.

The truth I speak of here is the knowledge and basic scientific and spiritual understanding of how the universal life energy seeks dynamic balance and correct flow through all things and how that affects us. The knowledge of this and the ability and intention to correct imbalance and blocked or misdirected energy flow makes up the truth of what sets us free. The holistic energy healing basic premise that all pain and suffering is due to an interruption of the balance and proper flow of energy has universal agreement. The methods and modalities to reestablish the proper dynamic balance and resolve the interruption to effect the proper flow, by their nature, bypass the debilitating issues of cause and effect thinking, rationalizing, competing opinions, right and wrong arguments, sin and punishment practices, and lies and stories as ways to finding or denying truth.

The Roots of Muscle Testing

It was Dr. George Goodheart who was the originator of Applied Kinesiology, the diagnostic procedure using muscle testing as the primary source method of feedback indicating how the body is functioning. If done correctly it could also indicate the best treatment for poor functioning. In the mid 60's Dr. Goodheart observed that a weak muscle could be treated and the strength immediately improved. From that observation his life became a search for other treatment methods that could improve muscle strength. In his search he realized that there were factors that could negatively affect the strength and functioning of muscles. Standard kinesiology was the study of motion, movement and muscle function, but what he was investigating was not a standard procedure. He found that the body would test strong, or "say yes" to the treatment or substances it needed and weak or "say no" to treatments and substances that were inappropriate. In the medical profession, this became a very effective therapeutic tool for physical and nutritional considerations in treatment.

Dr. John Diamond, Psychiatrist, who adapted applied kinesiology to his work which was largely influenced by preventive medicine, wrote in the *Journal of the International Academy of Preventive Medicine*, July 1977, pp. 97-99, "Applied Kinesiology may turn out to be the most therapeutic advance of this century! It has already revolutionized many practices including my own. I would venture to say that in the next few years it is going to cause tremendous changes in all branches of the healing professions open to change and improvement." This visionary statement has come into fruition.

Dr. Diamond went on to use muscle testing extensively in his holistic approach to health and wellness which included mental, emotional, spiritual and environmental factors along with physical and revolutionized preventative medicine with the philosophy and practice of what became Behavioral Kinesiology applying to all levels of being with an amazing range of applications. His book, *Your Body Doesn't Lie*, 1979 is a great read on this subject.

David Hawkins, M.D., Ph.D. in his landmark book, *Power vs. Force* explains further how the ensuing research and application and clinical kinesiology muscle testing has found widespread verification and use over the last 35 years. He explores the capacity of the human organism to differentiate at deep levels of awareness. He created the map of consciousness, an amazing scale for understanding the calibration of energy of emotions and all possible levels of human awareness. In my estimation, this is a must read.

The major advances that muscle testing offers is that it allows us to access the innate wisdom of the body/subconscious to hear firsthand what is wrong and what the body needs directly from the body. The amazing self-healing body is consulted as the expert energy and information, diagnostic and therapeutic tool it is. This is congruent with the basic premise of all healing that the body knows, heals from the inside out, is discriminating and with the right questions we can determine the origin of the problem and the best treatment as instructed by the unique and individual field consulted. The process of healing is observed and adjusted as shown to us by the body until the proper balance and flow of energy is reestablished.

How Do I Muscle Test?

This is a huge field of knowledge and applications with many nuances and considerations. You will be hearing more about Muscle Testing later, because it is a major supporting technique in healing of all kinds. The information offered here is meant to serve as learning awareness and understanding of the correlation of muscle testing and the flow of energy in accessing internal information. We will learn two kinds of Muscle Testing - testing with another person and self-testing. We will learn two variations within those categories and review cautions to remember when using energy testing.

Cautions First:

- Approach muscle testing with curiosity and open mind, in a safe and sacred space.
- If you are not grounded and centered and/or are emotionally or mentally upset, the testing will not work and may produce results opposite the truth. This is true of the person being tested and the person doing the testing.
- Do not use testing for major lifestyle changes.
- Do not use testing to determine another's emotions, actions or intentions or without their permission.

Some Good Uses for Muscle Testing:

- For holistic and energy therapy practitioners and therapists and doctors during treatment as a diagnostic tool.
- For energy psychology modalities, the treatment of allergies, applied and behavioral kinesiology and energy medicine treatment.
- Identifying and/or validating limiting beliefs
- Choosing (or not) a supplement use and dose
- Choosing between possible supplements
- Finding the origin of a problem
- Picking the best option of choices you have such as a breakout option at a conference, movie, menu selection, etc.
- Asking if a healing technique you have learned is best or appropriate for certain circumstances

Practicing self muscle testing alone or with someone else who wants to practice:

A. The Sway Test

1. Ground and center
2. Stand comfortably in an area free of distractions of any kind
3. Feet are shoulder width apart and hands comfortably hanging at your sides

4. You can close your eyes if you wish.
5. Notice your body is constantly adjusting with very slight movements.
6. Now make a positive, congruent statement and notice that your body will noticeably sway forward in less than 10 seconds
7. Go back to step four and five and neutralize your position
8. Now make a negative or incongruent statement and notice that your body will noticeably sway backwards.
9. Now just experiment with positive and negative words, ideas, feelings, etc.

Variations for self-testing:

B. O-ring Test:

1. Make a circle with the thumb and index finger of the same hand. Press only lightly.
2. Place the index finger of the other hand inside the circle and try to break the circle where the thumb and index finger meet.

C. Knee Test

1. Seated or standing raise one knee and push down on it with your hand. A "lock" in the hip joint is yes and an "unlock" is no.

Practicing energy testing with another person:

A. The Arm Test

1. Both ground and center
2. Ask the person if he/she has any shoulder problem or pain-If so, use the other arm. If both shoulders are painful use another way to test or you can surrogate test using another person or yourself as the surrogate and using self-testing.
3. Have the person stand with one arm out horizontal to the floor, hand in line with the arm and relaxed
4. Place your index and middle finger on the wrist of the extended arm and tell them you will have them say a statement and then you will apply light pressure on the arm and attempt to push it down. Tell them to resist and to try to prevent you from pushing their arm down.

5. Have the subject say their name as a sentence "My name is _____."
6. Pause a second and then push lightly and increasingly heavier for about three seconds. Use minimum force necessary
7. The shoulder should remain locked
8. Now repeat the test but this time have the subject say another name you give them that is not theirs. "My name is Isabel."
9. Pause a second and then push lightly and increasingly heavier for about 3 seconds. Use minimum force necessary
10. The shoulder should release and unlock

Now you can experiment with positive and negative thoughts and emotions and test the effect on the body. End on a positive note.

Variation for Arm Testing:

B. Arm down to side test

Have the arm position down to the sides and test by putting four fingers inside the wrist and pressing the arm away from the body.

Helpful Hints when energy testing:

• Remain neutral, keep your mind clear and calm and be respectful
• Do not smile or look into the subject's eyes
• Allow enough time for responses
• If the timing of questions and testing gets disjointed, start over
• Be sure you and the subject breathe deeply and stay hydrated – Actually this is always good advice!

NowOpp@MuscleTesting

To test the effect of negative and positive thoughts on the energy system with either self-testing or testing with another person:

• Select the type of muscle testing you will use.
• Take some deep breaths and be sure you are hydrated.

- Do a trial test saying " this is a yes" pause slightly and test-should test strong
- Do a trial test saying "this is a no" pause slightly and test – should test weak

(This is a simple test but muscle testing is complex with many factors. So if you get reverse of conflicting results, take a break, breath and hydrate and try again. Sometimes the subject is not testable for various reasons. When you get an accurate baseline test, then proceed)

- Now have subject think about something that bothers him/her a lot, pause and test – should test weak.
- Now have the subject allow that to go and replace it with something that always makes him/her very happy, pause and test – should test strong.

Variation:

You can practice muscle testing with a substance like a refined sugar cube. A person almost always tests negative/weak when holding the sugar cube in hand. Then replace it with an apple and test. People almost always test positive when holding an apple.

Have fun, learn and remember the cautions about muscle testing. For further study, Google "Muscle Testing"

There is no longer any reason to suffer or struggle.
In fact, it is a serious waste of time and energy.
It is now time to understand, rejoice,
Be peaceful, powerful and purposeful. Yes, but how? You ask?
You are finding out!

—Andrea 2009

Negative and Positive Belief — The building blocks of your Life Experience

Core negative life beliefs can be conscious or subconscious. They influence what we think of ourselves and our opinions and choices. They are not true, but because of experiences and/or other beliefs, we think they are true. They are detrimental to our health and well-being and can make our lives miserable and at the very least, limit our joy significantly.

Negative Life Beliefs	Positive Life Beliefs
I don't deserve love	I deserve love; I can have love
I am a bad person	I am a good (loving) person
I am terrible	I am fine as I am
I am worthless (inadequate)	I am worthy; I am worthwhile
I am shameful	I am honorable
I am not lovable	I am lovable
I am not good enough	I am deserving (fine/okay)
I deserve only bad things	I deserve good things
I cannot be trusted	I can be trusted
I cannot trust myself	I can (learn to) trust myself
I cannot trust my judgment	I can trust my judgment
I cannot succeed	I can succeed
I am not in control	I am now in control
I am powerless (helpless)	I now have choices
I am weak	I am strong
I cannot protect myself	I can (learn) to take care of myself
I am stupid (not smart enough)	I have intelligence (able to learn)
I am insignificant (unimportant)	I am significant (important)
I am a disappointment	I am okay just the way I am
I deserve to die	I deserve to live
I deserve to be miserable	I deserve to be happy
I cannot get what I want	I can get what I want
I am a failure (will fail)	I can succeed
I have to be perfect (please)	I can be myself (make mistakes everyone)
I am permanently damaged	I am (can be) healthy
I am ugly (my body is hateful)	I am fine (attractive/lovable)
I should have done something	I did the best I could
I did something wrong	I learned (can learn) from it
I am in danger	It's over; I am safe now
I cannot stand it	I can handle it
I cannot trust anyone	I can choose who to trust
I cannot let it out	I can choose to let it out

The Whole Truth of You

Negative Life Beliefs	Positive Life Beliefs
I do not deserve...	I can have (deserve)...
I cannot stand up for myself	I can make my needs known
I am different (don't belong)	I am okay as I am
I should have known better	I do the best I can (I can learn)
I am inadequate	I am capable
I am not safe	I am safe
I am unworthy	I am worthy
It's not okay to feel (show) my emotions	I can safely feel (show) my emotions
I am guilty	I am responsible
I am alone	I am encompassed
I am a victim	I am sturdy, strong
I am vulnerable	I am confident
I am incompetent	I am competent
I am misunderstood	I am understood
I am abandoned	I am rescued
I am betrayed	I am forgiving
I am sinful	I am virtuous
I am separated from God	I am united with God
I am unproductive	I am productive
I am unattractive	I am attractive
I am trapped	I am free
I am incapable	I am capable
I am confused	I am sound
I am a burden	I am enjoyable
I am used	I am valuable
I am unteachable	I can learn
I have no soul	I have a soul
I have no identity	I have an identity
I deserve pain	I deserve happiness
I deserve punishment	I deserve rewards
I deserve failure	I deserve success
I cause misfortune	I cause prosperity
I cause separation	I cause unity

Resource Guide: Negative and Positive Beliefs List by Gregory J. Nicosia, Ph.D., DCEP

The following NowOpps are three practice segments as part of one process. The three segments are: 1. Practice in muscle testing. 2. Clearing negative beliefs that may be inhibiting you. And, 3. Replacing the negative with a positive belief affirmation energetically, using the Universal Healing Heart Massage Technique. Take your time and follow the directions closely.

NowOpp@MuscleTestingForNegative Beliefs

This is a deductive process using muscle testing to find a negative belief you may or may not be aware of that is holding you back. Follow these steps:

1. Take one or two deep breaths and be sure you are hydrated, grounded and centered
2. Locate the negative life belief by using the negative and positive belief lists and muscle testing the following statements:

"My core negative life belief is on the first page" – if weak, go to the second page and test "My core negative life belief is on the second page"

3. When the page is established, muscle test the following statements:

"My core belief is on the top half of the page" – if weak, go test "My core belief is on the bottom half of the page"

4. When the top or bottom of the page is established, muscle test the following statements:

"It is in the top quarter" if weak, "It is in the bottom quarter." Then, "Top four or bottom four, top two, bottom two..." until you locate the belief statement that tests strong.

5. Then test the corresponding positive statement – It should test weak.

You have found your core negative belief. Notice your reaction and how you feel about it. You may or may not be surprised. Now move on to clearing it.

NowOpp@ClearingNegativeBeliefs

1. Take one or two deep breaths and be sure you are hydrated, centered and grounded
2. Using the Universal Healing Heart Circle to clear the negative belief, place the palm of one of your hands on the center of your chest, the heart chakra. Make a circle up towards the left shoulder and down and around up to the right shoulder back to where you started (that is clockwise if the clock is on your chest)
3. As you are circling your hand, say "Even though I believe I _____ (negative belief), I completely accept and love myself"(c.a.l.m.). Repeat this three times. Still circling your heart chakra, use the statements: "Even if I never get over believing _____ (negative belief), I completely accept and love myself, and I respect my feelings and ideas and thoughts about this belief and I completely accept and love myself"
4. Now take some deep breaths and be sure you are properly hydrated
5. Notice how you feel. What this does is release the interruption, so the energy can move and resolve. It enables you to be more neutral and calm about whatever the issue is
6. Now muscle test the negative belief. If strong, repeat the process. If weak, congratulations!

Now move on to replace the negative belief with the corresponding positive belief.

NowOpp@ReplacingNegativeBeliefs

1. Take one or two deep breaths and be sure you are hydrated, centered and grounded
2. Note the corresponding positive belief and use that statement for the following using the Universal Healing Heart Massage to replace the negative belief:
3. Place the palm of one of your hands on the center of your chest, the heart chakra. Make a circle up towards the left shoulder and down and around up to the right shoulder back to where you started (that is clockwise if the clock is on your chest)
4. As you are circling your hand, say "I know now that I _____(positive belief), and I completely accept and love myself" (c.a.l.m.). Repeat this three times. Still circling your heart chakra, use the statements: "Even if I feel I don't yet totally believe _____ (positive belief), I choose it over the negative belief and I completely accept and love myself, and I respect my feelings and ideas and thoughts about this belief and I completely accept and love myself." Or, "Even though I felt I didn't deserve love, I choose to feel deserving of love." And repeat it three times.
5. Now take some deep breaths and be sure you are properly hydrated.
6. This energetically replaces the negative belief. Notice how you feel.
7. Now muscle test the positive belief. If weak, repeat the process. If strong, congratulations!

Section Four

**Navigating Life as a Spiritual Energy
Being in a Physical Body**

The Nature of the Territory Called the Universe

I was destined to have the great fortune to travel the world (and other dimensions) over many years and for many reasons. I didn't realize at the time what was really happening. I didn't realize it would eventually be part of my destiny and life purpose as a healing educator. What I did notice and realize, but still not why, was that anywhere I would go, I would somehow end up with a local healer, experiencing and being taught how to do many different kinds of healing modalities. They acted like they knew me and charged me with the ability and responsibility to understand and to pass it forward.

Now when I look back on my life...particularly the last forty years, it has been a slow motion great matrix, filling in dots of experience and information to grant me the delight of an overall understanding and knowledge of healing possibilities and the resonance in which they take place. I laugh when I remember berating myself for not being able to specialize in something and do that one thing really well. What I realize now is I was specializing in what I really believe I was sent here to do.....integrate ancient and contemporary knowledge for teaching and healing myself and others in this astounding time in the history of life.

Prior to that realization, at one point of extreme doubt about what I was here for, my three very succinct gentlemen spiritual guides actually made one of their rare and brief visits to me and stated this:

"Pay attention to your sleeping dreams."

Two days later, their instructions applied clearly during a dream in which I was floating above the Earth, free of the force of gravity and noticing the many intricate, bright and colorful matrix configurations. At the time, I thought they were simply beautiful evolving colors and patterns, but then realized what I was seeing was the actual construction and movement of the life energy. I had been trained to ask what I was to learn from dreams which I did, and the Earth spoke in a loving and powerful way:

"Please help. See the patterns and make them seeable." I didn't know what patterns, what they meant or to whom I was to make them seeable, but I had learned to trust I need not know in that moment, and it would become clear when I needed to know. Mother

Earth's plea for help was permanently lodged in my heart and I woke up sobbing and grateful for the direction.

What I have come to understand is we live in a predictable numerical, geometric and impartial universe where all things are connected and all things are possible. The ultimate pattern is inclusive of all things. I had known this from my experiences in a spiritual, multicultural way, but the main understanding really came from the scientific views and theories that became available. Dr. Deepak Chopra is a stunning and eloquent spokesman and author for the understanding of the universal field in which we exist. The OldKnew views of the nature of reality are a result of science and spiritual quests coming together to the same conclusions:

There is no *external* or *internal*, nothing separate, only one field of existence of which we are each a microcosm of the macrocosm. We are like a drop of water in the ocean, made of the same stuff, unique and indispensible.

NowOpp@TheUnifiedField

Softly focus on the image on the next page by clairvoyant artist, Alex Grey. This is a depiction of how energy organizes in the Universal Mind/Consciousness/The Unified Field and "our" field. Get a sense of its complexity, endlessness, interrelatedness, predictability and harmony, and consider that this is your true nature as well.

Then contemplate the words in the chart on the next page and consider them accurate descriptions of you.

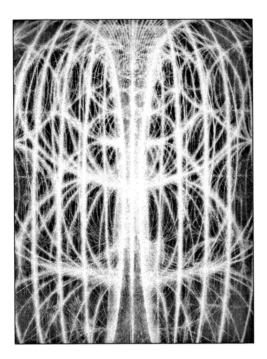

Image from *Sacred Mirror,* by Alex Grey

The Right Words to Describe the Real You

When we are asked to describe ourselves, we usually will relate our name, sex, roles, single, married, divorced, careers, stature, color of our eyes, color of our hair, where we went to school, who we look like, what we do or don't do, where we live, work, what we like, hobbies, accomplishments, fears, desires, hopes, dreams, etc. This never seems to really get to who we really are and most of those descriptions are transient. So who are we really?

Consider these words used to describe the unified energy field. Since we are a microcosm of the macrocosm of the universal field, these words describe our true nature. Look them over and nudge yourself to relate to the vibration the words hold. Begin to attempt to own this identity in an attempt to bridge the belief gap here.

Acceptance	All Knowing	Blissful	Clarity	Compassionate
Connectedness	Correctness	Divine	Ease	Evolutionary
Free	Fully Awake Within	Grace	Gratitude	Harmonious
Immortal	Infinite	Infinite Possibilities	Infinitely Creative	Infinitely Dynamic
Inherently Perfect	Inspired	Integrating	Joyous	Knowledge
Light	Limitless	Nourishing	Perfectly Balanced	Perfectly Ordered
Pure Awareness	Pure Knowledge	Pure Potential	Pure Silence	Pure Spirit
Playful	Purposeful	Sacred Warrior	Self-Healing	Self-Referral
Self-Sufficient	Truth	Unbounded	Unbounded Love	Unconditional Love
Unending	Un-manifest	Wholeness	Witness	Witnessed

The current leading scientific findings and the ancient texts are abundant and congruent with information and theory about the nature of the universe. In the resource section of this book, there are recommended reading resources on this subject for advanced learning.

Governing Influences of Our Souls' Journey

Out beyond ideas or wrong doing and right doing, there is a field.
I'll meet you there.

-Rumi

Using the combination of following my heart, grace and synchronicity, I found myself a part of the Chopra Center for Well-Being Staff. I had been there for over a year and a half at this point. I had begun as a volunteer and had now become a certified Chopra Center meditation teacher and Ayurvedic instructor. I loved being an educator and the new guest greeter, and teaching the orientation classes.

A requirement for working at the Chopra Center for Well-Being was to meditate with the staff every morning. I didn't think it got any better than this...until I was asked to take over as Program Director for the center and Director of the Global Network for Spiritual Success...a world-wide organization of study groups built around Deepak's wonderful book, *The Seven Spiritual Laws of Success.* I had been reading Dr. Chopra's books and listening to recordings of his lectures for quite some time. *The Seven Spiritual Laws of Success* particularly resonated with me and the natural approach and philosophies and books I had grown up with.

My Mother had a ninth grade education living in Greece as a child. When she came to America, she learned English reading cartoons and comic books. She was a passionate and discerning thinker. As a child, I was fortunate to have a wide variety of books available to me which helped to shape my thinking. My Mother has passed and I still have the exact books as treasures from my early years. I found most fairy tales scary and cruel, or silly, but for some reason which I wouldn't understand for years, however, I loved *Peter and the Wolf.*

My favorite "big person's" book was, *The Prophet,* by Kahlil Gibran, and I still read and quote it to this day. *Emerson's Essays* was a favorite of my Mom's and excerpts were often dinner table conversation. Thoreau was a close second, and I can remember thinking he was such a gentle, romantic and reassuring man...never having met him except through his writings. *As a Man Thinketh*, 1902 by James Allen, made perfect sense to me. I still have the treasured copy given to me by my Mother with this quote in her handwriting on the inside cover: "The thoughts that I think and the words that I speak cause only good in the world." *The Book of Life,* by Robe Collier, was inspiring and encouraging. I would read *One Hundred and One Famous Poems* and wonder why they were so famous. A pastime of mine for a while was my attempt to read the entire set of *The Great Books,* which I never did because I could not find relevance in them most of the time. I didn't know that at the time, I just thought it was because I was not a good reader, with which my second grade teacher agreed.

And so, early on I realized I was most drawn to writings that helped me understand the most unexplainable ways people think and act and the universe behaves. What I was learning in school only described behavior but not the "why's." Except for the opinions of the philosophers and psychologists quoted or mentioned briefly in my upper grade classes, most critical thinking was non-existent. It felt more like simply describing and classifying certain kinds of behavior and thinking rather than actually discovering the origins of the thoughts and of the behaviors and possibilities. I often thought the question, "Why do we just learn stuff someone already knows?"

So the *Seven Spiritual Laws of Success* filled a gap for me, because the why's of things were explained by seven basic laws of the universe. I found them intriguing and inspiring and expanding, and I was not the only one who felt that way. We started a study group on Monday nights at the Chopra Center and discussed one law a week. That went on for years. Soon the book began being published in different languages and is now published in over 50 languages. In the book was an invitation to start a study group and be part of the Global Network Study Groups. In a very short time, we had groups in 26 counties and we got volumes of mail. I had the great pleasure, along with my assistant and a volunteer staff, of processing the mail. We would categorize the questions and I would sit down with Dr. Chopra for an hour or so every month to obtain answers to questions asked. This experience showed me the common struggle, seeking and hope of all people.

The group of letters I was most moved by was the mail from prisoners. That book made such a difference for those who had not been able to follow the religious and manmade laws. They gave them hope and direction and a new way to look at themselves and at life and at society. This was a huge realization for me. Universal laws seemed freeing and inspiring. Religious and societal laws seemed limiting and punishing. In addition, all the societal and religious laws I had learned seemed distant and ancient and somehow not for me. It wasn't that I didn't believe they weren't correct. I just couldn't understand how I could be innately sinful and why there would have to be a law not to kill someone else or steal from them. It seemed that laws were made for the crimes and not for the people. What guided me were not the laws of the land or religious laws.

What guides you day-to-day in terms of choices, decisions, thoughts and actions? Do you lead a principle, value or purpose-centered life following natural laws, or perhaps a more regimented or conditioned, reactive or follow-the-rules life?

What I am proposing for our journey is a list of holistic living laws based on the energy and information patterns which govern us and the cosmos in which we find ourselves in this spectacular time in history. These timeless principles apply whether you are taking a scientific approach, a spiritual approach...a physical, emotional, psychological, philosophical, cultural or environmental approach. No matter what path appeals to you, if you know and apply these basic laws, you will be more able to understand what path is best for you, what is necessary to travel that path, and experience the desired growth and enlightenment you seek.

The integrated and synthesized laws from many influential sources during my lifetime have assisted me in making different and better choices. They offered a different line of thinking than I was accustomed to. The following selection of OldKnew laws are meant to be anchors throughout the book on our self-discovery journey. The philosophy and scientific bases of the laws will be mentioned as they are used as we address them.

And so, using the language of my heart and soul and experience, and with all due respect for all the influential sources from which they come, I offer to you what I feel to be the New World Universal Laws. An evolution in terms of focus and current knowledge expanded to be more applicable to our study of energy and vibration as it relates to our holistic approach and the description of the world today. I have compiled and integrated what I believe to be the most pertinent guidance, rules, and laws for these times. They have origins in many writings and experiences and include, *The Ten Commandments, The Seven Spiritual Laws of Success, Laws of Quantum Physics, Kundalini Yoga Teachings, LDS Word of Wisdom, Kabala Laws of Nature, Native American Natural Law, Energy Psychology Discovery Statement, The Old and New Testaments of the Bible, Right Use of Will Books, Anastasia Series, The Talmud, Power vs. Force, and Course in Miracles, The Prophet,* by Khalil Gibran, observing nature, latest scientific findings, just to mention a few, and of course, wisdom shared with me by the Divine Creator and my spirit helpers over time.

The following are the universal laws I feel we must know and understand as guidelines to harmonize and flow with the cosmos without sacrifice, struggle and with grace and ease during this intense transition and spiritual evolution demanded by the times. They have evolved with our understanding of how energy moves in our numerical universe. The reason they are important is they are new or altered points of reference to replace our previous bias and understanding no longer applicable that were based on the mechanized and institutional age we have just gone through.

These revised guidelines help train our brain to use new pathways of thinking to come to conclusions, resolutions and understandings that are nurturing and evolutionary. The understanding of these laws will come with the understanding of our own true identity as your awareness opens exponentially in our quest to unlock the truth, the whole truth and nothing but the truth.

For now, just read over, contemplate and read on with whatever understanding you glean. These will be our guideposts throughout the book.

Twenty - One Integrated New World Universal Laws - Guideposts for the Journey

> *When directed within, our attention introduces us to our true essence.*
>
> -Andrea Becky

When things seem wrong in our universe, it is because of interruptions of the field by improper or incorrect flow of the energy. The good news is improper and incorrect flow of energy can be understood, undone/healed and corrected, and the correct flow will resume. It is not corrected by manipulating, overpowering, and/or obliterating anything or anybody. It is done through understanding of how to resolve, disarm, and correct the interruptions and allow the natural and life-giving correct energy flow to resume. This is the basic premise of energy healing and it holds true for everything, everybody, the environment... all things manifesting and manifest.

Simply familiarize yourself with these laws and how they might assist in creating your joyous life. They will be referred to throughout the book in the practice section and personal practice section.

1. Our True Identity Is Pure Energy, Light and Information

Our true identity is luminous unbounded energy, vibration, information and light. We perceive, live and create life from our idea of who we are. We are much more than a body, mind and spirit. It is important that we have the sense of our true nature. It can only be known from introspection and experience. When we know our true identity, our true purpose, and true abilities, we can then meet our responsibilities with grace and ease and gratitude.

2. Attend To Self First

We are a sacred center in the Universe and of the same nature as the Universe, and we are responsible for care of Self first. The true experience and realization of our uniqueness and our unique gifts is necessary for us to be viable in life. It is a felt sense, not a concept. We must take care of ourselves first. This is not selfish, on the contrary, it would be selfish not to. For if we are not happy, healthy and balanced, we are unable to carry out our desires and share our gifts. No one else can live our lives and fulfill our destiny.

3. Everything is Energy and Vibration

Everything is energy and vibration and can be measured and calibrated. Once unseen and unknown and mysterious, the universal energy was a mystery. In our digital world with our highly technical scientific methods, we can now "see" energy, measure it and calibrate it in terms of compared vibration. We now know that negative thoughts, actions, emotions and deeds, calibrate under 200 on a scale of 1000. Positive thoughts, actions, emotions and deeds, calibrate higher. Enlightenment/pure consciousness calibrates above 700. In order to evolve spiritually, we must avoid negativity.

4. All is One/Nothing is Separate

There is now a beginning and no end. Philosophic discussions about the beginning of the Universe are basically useless. There is no cause and effect. There are only the effects and results of our thoughts, desires, emotions and choices. There is just a continuous cycle of cycles that appears to change. This premise can only be felt in a state of high consciousness and cannot be rationalized. So the question, "Which came first, the chicken or the egg?" can never really be answered.

5. Like Bonds with Like/Opposites Attract

You bond with like energy, you attract opposite energy, which seems like it is like energy. But more than likely it is something that you think completes you. Without an awareness of your true identity and clarity about your purpose, you will have difficulty knowing the difference.

6. Truth allows Truth

If you will give the gift of your authenticity/ your truth, you free others to do the same. That allows the life energy to flow correctly and for truth to live and nurture you and others. How we live, we become.

7. All Energy is Available Everywhere

By its very nature, energy is everywhere and exists with no time and no space. All energy is accessible by choice, constant, pure potentiality, continuous and simultaneously giving and receiving. Giving and receiving is the same continuum. You must give to receive and receive to give.

8. Attention Enlivens

Where we put our attention becomes strengthened and more alive. Choose to put your attention on only that which you desire to live in your life. Also, attention does not respond to "no" or "don't" or "never." It only responds to positive choice.

9. All Has An Effect and Consequence for All

For every impulse, thought, word and action, there is an effect and consequence to all. This is Karma. It is not punishment or reward, just the continuous flow of energy to and from the source of the impulse, thought, word or action.

10. Intention is the Universal Driving Force

Intention, conscious or unconscious, is the originator and perpetuator of all things. It is the driving force of all energy and manifestation. The problem lies in whose intention it is and what lies behind the intention. Is it divine intention or mundane intention? Is it for the higher good of all, or not?

11. In Context, Truth is Absolute

We know that truth has been considered relative. What is true for me may not be true for you. However, there is universal truth (correctness) that is indicated by the correct flow of the life force. This can now be measured with high tech instruments and with muscle testing within the context of the situation, and truth in that context is absolute. So I can know energetically what is absolutely true (correct) within the context of certain circumstances.

12. **The Unknown is Knowable**

   What was previously known as unknown is now known. There is still what is considered to be unknown waiting to be known. We have proven that the unknown is knowable.

13. **How the Brain is Used Affects the Way It Functions**

   How you use or don't use your brain affects how your brain will function. This is a major neurological discovery of our times, the neuroplasticity of the brain, frees us to enhance our brain function by choosing how we use our brain and for what.

14. **The Times Demand Compassion**

   Understand with compassion or you will misunderstand the times. There is nowhere to go and nowhere to hide and we are all doing the best we can. Only compassion will allow us to evolve as quickly as we must now. Compassion is not a concept; it is a state of being.

15. **Vibrate Your Path.**

   Vibrate the cosmos with a clear image and pure intent, and it will clear a path for you. We are now in an era of feeling our reality. The cosmos responds to clear and conscious images and pure single intent. Covert or competitive intent will be lost in the ethers.

16. **Recognize and Remember the Other Person is You.**

   We live in a reflective universe. In compassion and clarity of purpose, recognize that the other person is mirroring some aspect of you. Ask yourself what you need to learn.

17. **Pure Potentiality is Constant and Continuous**

   Source energy is constant and continuous. It is only our states of being that make it seem otherwise. To access pure potentiality, we must maintain constancy and balance.

18. **You Must Feel to Heal**

   We must become fluent in the language of vibration/ feeling our reality. This takes place at a very deep level. It is necessary to practice living at that deep level with grace and ease. If we do not, we will get lost in the negativity of our condition. We cannot think our way to enlightenment.

19. There Is A Way Through Any Problem

In a solution-based state of being, there is a way through any problem. It is gratitude, forgiveness, allowing, accepting, surrender, trust and being, not doing or controlling, that creates desired results. Enough said.

20. Remain in Consciousness

We are not in control of anything except choosing our state of being and where, when and how we step into or out of the stream of conscious. Enough said.

21. Serve Others

All life has a common purpose: manifest and express consciously your deepest driving desire for life using your unique gifts and abilities in service to others.

NowOpp@LifePurpose

Take some deep breaths and relax. Direct your attention inward and ask your higher self, "What are my unique gifts?" Get to know yourself at the level of your Soul and what you love.

And now on to more knowledge that expands your awareness beyond right and wrong...

The Fourteen Keys to Transformation, Creation and Manifestation

When will you realize that there is nothing that you need that you don't already have except the direct experience of there is nothing you need that you don't already have?

-Ken Keyes, *Handbook to Higher Consciousness*

The following are the keys to the knowledge, awareness and experience that continually create your reality. Properly used, they lead to the true experience of who you are and why you are here and living your authentic joyous life. You own these keys now. You may not be aware of their power, know they belong to you, or may have never thought of them in the ways we will be using them. Just familiarize yourself with them and the brief working definitions and characteristics given and you will be using them differently just from that awareness. They are the keys that unlock your joy and create your extraordinary joyous, healthy and exquisite life! This is a fourteen-step Now/Opp to understand the energy of each key. Read, feel and take a deep breath between each key.

1. **Perception - The Reality Creator**

   Our perceptions and the way we think and relate create our reality. Problems originate with perceptions that are subconscious and or conditioned or thought of as the truth when they are not. We form thoughts, judgments and beliefs based on our perceptions and many of them did not originate within us. If your current reality is not satisfactory, look first at your perception and the supporting beliefs that make it unsatisfactory and be open to new perceptions of the problems. So open discerning and non-judgmental perception is the goal.

   The most devastating misperception is our perception of ourselves as limited and finite. It affects everything we do every day. That is why the basic premise of healing ourselves and others must begin with us and a true perception about our true infinite identity.

   ...breathe...

2. **Attention – The Life Giver**

   Attention activates whatever it is drawn to. The more we put our attention on something, the more alive it becomes. This is apparent when we dwell on something. After a while it seems like whatever we are dwelling on is dwelling on us and we can't stop. Also, attention doesn't understand commands like don't, no, none, or never. For example, if I say "Don't pay attention to page 336 in this book".....I know where your attention is right now! I am sure you have experienced statements like, "I will never drink too much/eat too much sugar/lie/buy too much/ again" never going very far. So consciously choosing where we put our attention and why is the goal.

   ...breathe...

82

3. Intention – Fuel of Manifestation

Intention is the fuel for our ideas, desires, goals, and projects. The problems with this start with the fact that intention can be conscious or subconscious, reactive, denied or disguised or not pure in many ways. So the fuel goes to waste or starts a fire we can't put out. Developing clarity of intention and learning the power of intention and consciously setting and projecting intention is the goal here.

...breathe...

4. Experience – The Memory Teacher

Our lives are simply a series of experiences. They are the culmination within which our thoughts, ideas, choices, actions or awareness (or lack of) play out. Most think experiences just happen to us. In actuality, learning to choose what we experience is part of a major skill in creating a joyous life. Experiences are stored in our subconscious and build upon each other, become our believed life story, and the more they repeat, the more we think they are "the truth" of who we are. In fact, they are only what has happened to us. Consistently creating desired experiences is the goal here. To do this well, we need to know ourselves at the level of the Soul and have a clear sense of our Soul's purpose, which is one of the desired effects of this book, for the trick is that experience shows us who we are like nothing else can.

Experience is a complex dynamic. It involves free will, perception, discernment, feeling, attitude, karma, self-image and self-knowing. Experience imprints knowledge and awareness in our field. We must choose and process our experiences with the best wisdom we have. If our heart is not engaged, we can make poor choices that have poor results. Experience is the crux and a measurement of transformation, for as we transform and expand our consciousness, our experiences change. We must experience to truly understand. We are not our experiences.

...breathe...

5. Awareness – The Door Opener

Awareness is complex in that it depends on the detection and clearing of obstacles to awareness, like negativity, negative beliefs, emotional turmoil, like fear, anger, hate, resentment, jealousy, sadness, and states of anxiety, depression, grief, frustration, less than, abandonment, betrayal. These obstacles, when identified and resolved, lead to greater awareness. It also depends on the conscious seeking of greater awareness through spiritual practices, curiosity, study, research, inquisitiveness, acceptance, compassion, gratitude and willingness to be out of your comfort zone. The goal here is to value the unknown and unexperienced and consistently question what is, why it is and how it could be different.

...breathe...

6. Breath – Universal Life Force

Our constant companion, and at our beckoned call, the breath is our most primary and immediately accessible transformation tool. The breath is akin to the very life force and for every state of being there is a breath pattern reflecting the quality of the experience. If we do not like our state of being, we can change it by changing the breath pattern.

Pranayam: the conscious study and healing practice of using the breath is an empowering multi-level and immediate key to health and well-being on all levels, true identity, and sustainable transformation. Conscious use of the breath brings a sense of higher consciousness and a deep heightened awareness to our automatic breathing.

...breathe...

7. Sensation – The Awakener

Sensation, especially from an unknown source, is the awakener. It brings awareness to information and/or issues we are more than likely not aware of. The biggest mistake we make with sensation is lack of awareness, immediately judging it as good or bad, not allowing it or having time to be informed by it. The goal here is to be open to possibilities and not have to know immediately what the sensation "means." This is an intuitive practice.

...breathe...

8. Emotion – The Informer

Ah, emotion, the most misunderstood energy of all. There is a great deal of misinformation, judgment and fear around

84

emotions. The greatest tragedy, in my opinion, is all the time, effort and money we spend not to feel, ranging from pharmaceuticals to addiction, denial and outdated coping mechanisms. Emotional energy is meant to be energy in motion, the informer and the voice of the Heart. Emotions try to inform us of our good choices and not so good choices. The only bad emotion is a stuck emotion. The research tying suppressed emotion to disease is startling and undeniable.

The goal here is to learn to deal safely with feeling and being correctly informed by emotions. That is one of the specialties of energy healing! We are not our emotions.

...breathe...

9. Imagination – The Igniter

When used consciously, imagination is the path out of "stuckness," the problem-solving machine, the creator. When used as an escape or carelessly or reactively, it is the destroyer.

It is an indispensible key for transformation. It allows us to connect the dots virtually as needed in this largely virtual world. The goal here is the development of conscious imaging for healing and creating the joyous life we so desire. We are not our imagination.

...breathe...

10. Memory – The Reminder

Memory is our virtual connection to all life and dimensions, conscious and subconscious. Memory does not stand alone. It is necessarily connected to images, people, things, places, time, emotion, thought, touch, sight, sound, smell and taste and other memories, and those can be the triggers that bring a memory back. Recalling memories has a physiological affect. If the memory is pleasant, the body responds with pleasure. If the memory is painful, the body responds with that pain. If the memory is neutral (consider it more like just a fact), the body will just acknowledge it, re-record it and move on. The important thing to remember here is that memory is cellular. The goal is to get back to the memory of our true identity, We are not our memories.

...breathe...

11. Movement – The Integrator

Every move we make affects our entire field of energy. The body is designed to move and is constantly seeking dynamic balance on all levels of our being, even when we are physically still. Movement, like the breath, can be consciously used as a therapy. When writers and artists and project managers come to me because they feel blocked and unproductive, I prescribe movement of some kind to them. It works every time. Walking and breathing with intention, dancing of all kinds, martial arts of all kinds, organized fitness classes, like Nia and Zumba, home video workouts, are all examples of the movement available to us. Intention and action is all it takes. Thinking does not work in these circumstances, as I am sure you know. There will be more about movement later in this section.

Until then...

NowOpp@FluffYourAura

Any movement we make causes a shift in our balance and awareness. The Martial Arts like Chi Gong, Tai Chi, Tae Kwon Do, Aikido, and Karate, are based on consciously moving energy for protection, opening and correct flow.

A good exercise with similar intent, that will refresh and invigorate you, I call "Fluff Your Aura."

- Stand comfortably with feet shoulder-width apart, or you can be seated with no obstacles to arm movement
- With your palms up, begin making alternating upward movements all around your body as if you were trying to keep a beach ball in the air for about a minute
- Now with both arms, begin making figure eight movements in front of the body and allowing your body to sway with them for about one minute
- Now place the palms on the thighs, take a deep breath and close your eyes for about a minute
- Take a deep breath and relax and open your eyes slowly and feel refreshed and invigorated

---

12. Creativity – The Innovator

Many say to me, "I'm just not creative" and ascribe creativity to those in the creative arts; however, our creativity is how we change ourselves, our lives and our environments. Without creativity, we are subject to things as they are and other's creativity and a reactionary life. It is the process of taking what we know, adding to, deleting, modifying, re-associating and/or rearranging its meaning and/or order to create a new meaning, use or function. It is the function of desire, the imagination, memory and the creative mind – uncommon thinking. The phrase, "Necessity is the mother of invention," has ancient roots. A good example of this is someone who is lost in nature with nothing and has to find a way to survive with nothing; stay warm or cool, deal with an injury, find food and water, build a fire, find the way out or home. Ideally, this process is a good way to approach our problems and difficulties and find resolution and solutions in innovative ways. We are not our creativity.

...breathe...

13. Silence – Where the Truth Is

Silence allows pure potentiality to abound and diminishes the distractions that keep us from our true reality. This is why most healing practices will involve silence and/or sound and movement that silence the mind to reach silence. This silence is stillness within that entrains with the silence of cosmic consciousness. It is a sweet, fully-nurtured and protected state of being you may have experienced. The goal is to experience that at will. That is why we seek the knowledge, awareness and experience to do so. That is the reason for this book. We find ourselves in silence.

...breathe...

14. Reflection – The Reality Checker

Reflection is simply feedback energy and information. We have the reflection that our senses give us in our waking state, the reflection of seemingly no reflection when sleeping, the reflection of sleeping dreams, and we at some level think that is our reality and we set about creating or changing those reflections to meet our desires. But that is an incomplete story of our existence.

What reflects reality to us is what I call the "all that is continuously one, timeless and formless, limitless, unbounded, and with no inside or out, no top or bottom, beginning or end, unable to be separate, the unknown that becomes known." This cosmic/pure consciousness...the source of all things... pure potentiality, that which expresses and expands through us and this is our true reality. Self-reflection is a most powerful tool to develop the ability to identify and access cosmic consciousness. Nature demonstrates the energy of oneness, and all fourteen keys, when used with awareness, unlock the door to this reality. We are not our reflection.

...breathe...

Speaking the Nine Languages of You As You Travel— Are You Fluent?

You are what your deep, driving desire is. As your desire is, so is your will. As your will is, so is your deed. As your deed is, so is your destiny.

-Brihadaranyaka Upanishad

How did I know that? Since no one else was asking how I knew the things I knew, and actually thought I was making it up, I began to ask myself how I knew the things I knew. The problem was, as soon as I would begin to think about it, I would begin to question if it was true myself (although with most of me, I knew it was). That most of me that knew was my felt sense state of awareness. And so, at a very young age, I realized that there was an energy/feeling/sensation that informed me. And those qualities would turn into worldly things like ideas, imaginary friends, knowingness and facts about ultimate truths. Needless to say, that was not what I was being taught in school, although what I was learning was showing me the difference and helping me to know myself and the world by comparison.

Other great teachers were society and culture. I was born in Salt Lake City, Utah in St. Michaels Hospital, of Greek decent and Greek Orthodox religious beliefs. By the time I was four, I realized that I was in an extreme minority in the Salt Lake area with that background. I didn't think of it that way, but was aware that every neighbor and friend in our neighborhood (my universe at that time) was not Greek and not Greek Orthodox, but Mormon and of northern European decent. I wondered how and why that happened. On Sundays, I would go the Greek Church and Greek School with my Mom. I loved sitting on the aisle, where the aroma of the incense was strongest, hearing the priest sing in Greek (which I did not understand) and looking at all the familiar icons of The Eye of God, Mother Mary, Jesus and Saints and Angels. The energy there infused me with warmth and security and an expansive feeling. I would see my aunts and uncles and cousins most of which lived in other parts of town, and there would often be festive wedding, baptism and funeral celebrations in the hall next to the church. I can still take myself there with the aroma of cigars and bourbon and dancing to Greek music, the most wonderful delectable pastries the women had been baking all week, and the sounds and sights of whole families from new born babies to the oldest of great, great grandmas and grandpas. This gave me a sense of belonging and community. That felt complete and correct.

At the same time, the neighbors and neighborhood friends would go to the LDS ward. I didn't know what that was like and my playmates never talked about it, I never asked, and they never asked me about my church. That felt a bit incomplete and empty.

Because of my felt awareness learning, I learned that a correct full safe feeling was a good feeling and an empty, unspoken, unknown feeling was somehow wrong or undesirable. That was good enough for me, but as time went by, I noticed that people would talk about feelings, they would refer to nice feelings as good and not nice feelings as bad. And the conversations turned to right and wrong with overtones of blame and ignorance, comparison and competition, and I began to learn the underpinnings of prejudice and bias. I began to learn and experience the gaps of understanding in society and a culture of separation. That did not feel good.

So I learned to rely more and more on my reasoning and less and less on my feelings, as I set upon the path to figure out these circumstances and my place in it all. I began to lose fluency in my felt sense and at the time this was all happening for me, we had phones that were stationary and plugged into the line in the wall. We had shared lines called party lines. Our belief and perception

89

was that information (voiced words) traveled along telephone wires. What I didn't know cognitively and was not aware of, was Universal Energy and the way that energy and information flows continually everywhere and how to tap into it reliably and intentionally. We are fortunate now to have the direct knowledge and experience that energy is everywhere, and we can access it from anywhere with our "search engine technologies" and our "search engine abilities" and how that applies to your true sense of yourself.

What Languages do You Speak? Or Don't Speak? Or Have Forgotten?

Can you speak the languages of you? For the most part, we speak to ourselves in words...some nice and most not so nice, and the many other languages have been silenced. We define and explain ourselves with words, titles, roles, categories, gender, race, skin color. Where has that gotten us? When we begin to get an idea of our true limitless and whole identity, we realize we need to recognize and speak many languages. Words are only the language of our rational ego minds which tend to be repetitive, divisive and circular in energetic nature which, compared to other languages of ours, is rather limited. Have you ever found yourself thinking and saying the same things to yourself and others every day, or having the same problems over and over? This is a sign of limited and incorrect self-communication and self-knowledge and self-identity.

Learn to be aware of the universal language of life...VIBRATION, sometimes referred to as SILENCE...it is our true first language. We must become fluent in the languages of us to know our true Identity and live in expanded conscious awareness sometimes called Bliss or Enlightenment. All the languages we will explore now transmit energy and information necessary for us to process our lives correctly. If we cannot understand the language of the energy and information message, it can get misplaced and skewed, and the possibilities of a positive outcome may be lost in reaction.

Example 1: I feel hurt. That makes me angry. It's his/her fault. I resent him/her. He/she should....

Example 2: I feel blissful. I don't even know why. This is not normal. I must be crazy. I don't know who I am when I feel this way.

From the effects of negative influences, social and/or religious morays, negative experiences, we can lose our ability to speak the languages of us out of fear, trauma, rules spoken and unspoken or teachings of being silent, non-assertive, or feelings of inferiority or inappropriateness. All of what I have just mentioned are areas of life that energy healing can correct and resolve quite reliably, which is necessary to unlock your joy and create your joyous life. It is imperative that you become familiar with the languages of you and in which ones you are fluent, have forgotten, or perhaps, never learned.

The Nine Languages of a Joyous Life Master

1. The Language of the Rational Mind (Ego) – Thoughts/Words
2. The Language of the Higher Self – Intuition
3. The Language of the Subconscious – Memories
4. The Language of the Creative Mind – Images
5. The Language of the Body – Sensation
6. The Language of the Heart – Emotions
7. The Language of the Will – Impulse/Action
8. The Language of the Soul – Desire
9. The Language of The Source of All Things – Consciousness

All of these languages are interrelated and running all the time. The ones we can hear and translate are the ones upon which we put our attention...or the ones that are being ignored or unheard and finally get so loud, we cannot ignore them any longer and we find ourselves is some crisis and that is all we can hear or think about... again. The ones we don't know get us the same results we get when we are traveling without a translator in a region and don't know the language.

Neuroscience has shown that every one of these languages has an instant and direct substantive effect on our bodies, minds and spirits. Each experience of each language releases information substances with our field ranging from energetic configurations, flow or blocks to hormones, peptides and neurotransmitters. If the experience is negative, the substances are detrimental, if the experience is uncharged or neutral, homeostasis is maintained, if the experience is positive, the effects are beneficial.

Just think about it for a moment. How do you feel after a good laugh? How do you feel after being very angry or hurt? How do you feel on an average "inconsequential" day? That is your body telling you if that was a positive, neutral or negative experience. Of course, this is a simplification for we are complex beings in a complex environment, but for the purpose of understanding and in reality, we only exist in the moment.

Thanks to the yogis, rishis, seers and scientists, what we know now is we are capable of tuning into any language at any given time and speak it fluently if we have experienced the language and are balanced. Our conditioning, learning experiences, individual and collective thought belief and religious, political and social biases keep us from speaking fluently all languages of our existence.

- The first key to fluency is awareness of the languages.
- The second key is to create enough of the universal language of "The Now Silence" in your life.
- The third key is to listen in the Now Silence where these communications can be felt/ heard and spoken fluently.

1 - THOUGHTS/WORDS -
The language of the Rational Mind/Ego

Words have defined meaning; however, the vibratory quality of a word and how it is said or thought carries even more meaning. It is the conditioning and the states of being of the person thinking or speaking the word and of the person hearing the word that determine the power of the word and the message. The grouping and sequencing of words also affect meaning. And words actually end up being conditional and relative and easily carry double-meaning. Intent, conscious and subconscious affect the meaning as well. It is the subjective reaction to the word that really carries the meaning. So words, even though they are the major communication form in our culture, are a somewhat inadequate form of communication. We refer to this with phrases like "one picture is worth a thousand words," or "silence is golden" or "actions speak louder than words" or "talk about it or do it" or "talk is cheap." But words do have their place and have been a boon historically for human evolution, for education and communication, and I would have a hard time writing this book without them. Just suffice to say they are possibly limiting and overrated and/or overused to run our lives. It is good to have a way with words and to be well-spoken, but there is so much that depends on a deeper awareness than the mind and simply being literate. And the awareness of what is not being spoken and/or written sometimes has greater meaning. We are not the words used to describe us.

Thoughts are our interpretation of whatever comes into our awareness. The nature of the thoughts, again, depends upon our state of being and conditioning and brain function. Unfortunately, our precognitive biases and exterior and object referral tendencies make most of our thoughts and judgments...identifying, classifying, quantifying and qualifying. When we feel/sense/remain neutral before we think...we are more likely to assess a person, place, thing or incident more accurately. In addition, if we are reactive in our demeanor and act quickly or "without thought," more like, "without feeling," we are more likely to regret our actions except in some cases of "instinctual right action."

Another quality of thoughts that is limiting is a very large percentage of daily thoughts tend to be "automatic" and repetitive and result in automatic and repetitive behavior which can be desirable, however, is usually not. It is common to think we are our thoughts, and our thoughts and actions or behaviors become so enmeshed, they are indistinguishable. In this case, it is more important to be aware of what came before and after the thought. If we are in a "mindless automatic thinking state," this is nearly impossible and becomes a detriment when dealing with thoughts and behaviors that are problematic, like those when dealing with addiction.

Asking the rational brain to help with emotional issues is like vacuuming the family room with a lawn mower, it seems to work okay, but does a lot of damage. Remember that the rational mind/left hemisphere of the brain is like a linear processor and works like a computer in a linear way, in sequence, depends on details, from details to the whole, and works in the way it has been programmed. It identifies, categorizes, defines, describes, compares, quantifies, organizes, selects facts that agree, breaks down the present moment into manageable bits of information, and weaves all the available information into a very believable, verifiable story. It is imperative for academic pursuits, to-do lists, balancing your check book and planning your calendar and getting around town, among a multitude of other things, and depends on words and numbers to express information.

It can become distracting, interruptive and annoying if not used correctly and will talk incessantly. Another problem is it defines us with titles, adjectives, affirmations and/or defamations, which may seem to be true, but keep us from the realization of our true identity.

The main problem with the rational mind or left hemisphere of the brain is we are so used to it running our lives, and we ask it to do things it cannot do...give us the experience of our true identity.

In order to be who we really are, our authentic selves, we must cultivate discerning, critical, mindful creative thinking patterns as the language of our ego, and speak all the languages of who we really are. We will address this in the healing practices section of the book. For now, remember, we are not our thoughts, we are not our behaviors, and we are not our titles or roles.

2 - INTUITION - The Language of the Higher Self

Intuition is mysterious. It is information received without reasoning, a feeling, hunch... Carl Jung said intuition is "...irrational and information arrived at through the subconscious."

Regardless of how intuition is described, it is information that cannot be validated in the way reasoning or factual information can. Intuition is often not validated except by a deep knowing and that is often not validated. So there is a great amount of trust and not having to know and bypassing the rational mind involved in developing the language of the Higher Self.

I believe I was born with intuitive skills because I cannot remember not having them, and have experienced past lives in which I had intuitive skills. However, I can remember abandoning and/or forgetting those skills to get along in an environment that was threatened by intuitive ability and knowledge.

What I have learned, is building confidence in intuitive powers involves calming the mind and raising conscious awareness to feel secure in the knowing that comes through intuitive channels. Calming the mind also expands the ability to access intuitive knowledge intentionally and beyond what you can even imagine and reduce the randomness of the nurturing flow of the gift of intuition.

We are not our intuition; however, it is an excellent source of clues about our true identity.

3 - MEMORIES - The Language of the Subconscious

We know now, thanks to the physicists, neuroscientists, and kinesesiologists, that every cell in our body has memory capability. And in fact, our gut cells have more memory capability than brain cells. Candace Pert, a noted neuroscientist and author of *Molecules of Emotion*, also has a wonderful lecture called, *Your Body is Your Subconscious*, in which she states that all memory is stored in the body, non-judgmentally, neutrally stashed and can be called upon *intentionally* and/or *unintentionally* through various triggers.

All memories are stored in the cells of the body which as we have learned, make up the subconscious. Some memories feel conscious and others are stored away and seemingly forgotten, guarded, repressed. The energy of all memories affects us in many ways, pleasant, neutral and unpleasant.

The emotions, images, thoughts and beliefs that make up the memories become as real again as the memories become activated, even if the event that produced the memory took place at a much earlier date. Not only that, but every one of the 75,000,000,000 cells that make up each of our bodies are all intelligent cells, and the remembering of the event or series of events that created the memory makes it all real again and can affect your body the same way it was affected in the first place.

Actually, this is what a fair amount of energy healing is about. Healing interruptions in the field and restoring neutrality to a charged situation so the person can resolve unpleasant effects of some life experiences and gain peace and understanding. We are not our memories.

For our purposes, I would like to make a distinction between the terms subconscious and unconscious because they are often used interchangeably, which can be confusing. The subconscious is a field of consciousness that we have previously thought inaccessible except through dreams, psychotherapy, hallucination and hysteria, to name a few circumstances. In the holistic energy healing way of thinking, so beautifully described by neuroscientist Candace Pert, Ph.D. in her audiobook, *Your Body is Your Subconscious Mind,* it is a cellular-based impartial recording of all that has ever happened to you consciously or unconsciously and the entirety of the experience of your soul is stored in your subconscious. The unconscious is a state of being in which one is not being aware of something.

Research scientists and doctors have repeatedly failed to locate the areas of the subconscious and memory in the brain. Sigmund Freud, neurologist and founding father of psychoanalysis, interestingly enough was one of the first to determine it is very difficult for us to know ourselves because we are made up of our conscious and unconscious or pre-conscious selves. Since he believed we were motivated primarily by sex and survival, he ascribed the suppression and repression of those primal drives to the unconscious/subconscious. Over time, this has attributed to the fear and reluctance to explore the subconscious, and in my opinion, has restricted important self-awareness and self-knowing at the soul level. Many have thought we would be horrified to find the truth of who we really are because we have thought we are our subconscious. We are not our subconscious.

Subconscious or unconscious memories or experiences are often the source of difficulties in the conscious world. The really good news is holistic practices and energy healing methods, therapies and protocols can and do find and resolve those origins. The healing is profound, sustainable and somewhat unbelievable at times. In many cases, the high percentage and permanence and quickness of healing and resolution creates a big belief gap between this new treatment reality and traditional treatment methods. However, the experience and the results are almost always undeniable. Suffice it to say, I look at the subconscious as a wonderland of healing possibilities.

4 - IMAGES - The language of the Creative Mind

The creative mind/right brain hemisphere speaks in images, and things that speak to the five senses – color, texture, smell, sound, pictures. It is a holistic processor. It begins with all possibilities or the big picture where all is one, and it is a more random associative pattern or matrix processor. Sequential thoughts are random and the creative/right hemisphere is attuned to intuited knowledge and thinking in the present moment. It creates an overview with conclusions rather than seeking the details and deductive processes of the rational/left hemisphere. It complements the rational mind in that it processes the subtleties of information such as tone of voice, facial expressions and body language. It is also more sensitive to double-meaning, incongruence and the complex energy dynamics of any given situation.

The main problem with creative mind is it is often underdeveloped particularly in western cultures and societies and/or underused or overrun by the critical nature of the rational mind. Its ability to take in information and think in a holistic way is often diminished by the over-conditioned or rationalization dominance of our rational mind left hemisphere and/or the inability to express the information in words.

The creative mind processing pattern is very helpful in our quest to know ourselves at a deep level because of the free association in the field of pure potential. It enables us to access experience and information <u>outside the box</u> more readily. Also, we know that physical movement activates and strengthens the right hemisphere processing. We are not our creative mind; however, it is an extremely helpful language leading to the experience of our true identity.

5 - SENSATION -The Language of the Body

From the ancient seers and sages to the modern scientists we have gleaned literally unbelievable information about the body, mind and spirit. The body is literally the most amazing creation in all of creation. In each moment, countless processes are being carried out automatically at the subconscious level by the innate wisdom of the body continually seeking homeostasis and adjusting to the continual changing dynamic of the unified field in which it has manifested and very efficiently managing seventy five trillion cells that make up this amazing phenomenon we live in. Spiritually and scientifically what we know is we are connected to all things through our unequaled and unprecedented detection system – with our chakras (energy power centers), meridians (energy channels), and biofield (the totality of our vibrational electromagnetic light and energy makeup).

The language of the body is sensation. It signals harmony and flow and/or discord and blockage on any level it may be occurring – physical, mental, emotional, spiritual and environmental.

The problem begins when we do not or cannot hear the language of the body. The problem is exacerbated by the incorrect translation of the language of the body and/or overriding because of misunderstanding about the body or with our precognitive beliefs and/or egoic pursuits.

The body (individual field of existence) is our Sacred home in the Universe. An understanding of the true nature of the body and a heightened ability to communicate with the body is imperative for the path to extraordinary health and an exquisite life. The therapies and technologies in the healing practices section of the book are largely body centered to develop the understanding and heightened body awareness necessary to succeed on this healing path. We are not our bodies.

6 - EMOTIONS - The Language of the Heart

Emotions are the great 24/7 informers that work with the nervous system to send very important messages. I believe emotional energy is the most misunderstood language and the most censored, medicated and the silenced source of suffering, discomfort, inflammation and disease in the body and the tragedy and heartbreak of abuse and/or of what could have been.

Emotions are categorized as good and bad, acceptable and unacceptable, when really the only bad or unacceptable emotion is a repressed, numbed or stuck emotion. If we speak the language, the emotional energy itself is a gift and informs us of correct and/or incorrect thoughts, feelings and actions. The problem is when we don't speak the language of the heart, then it is the mind and/or ego or misinformed will that interprets the message and that puts us on the proverbial emotional roller coaster.

Literally billions of dollars are spent each year in the attempt not to feel pain and/or emotion and the critical messages are lost. Pharmaceutics, addictions of all kinds...food, drugs, alcohol, sex, shopping, violence, and excess anything, renders the emotional energy useless but does not free it, and the informational message festers and waits for another opportunity to be heard.

The new technologies offered in this book enable a safe, healthy empowering and sustainable way to deal with the most debilitating of emotional energy. The emotional fitness process is a process of self knowledge, improved health, communication and relationship and authenticity. We are not our emotions.

7 - IMPULSE/ACTION - The Language of the Will

The thing that separates us from all other living things is Free Will: the ability to choose for ourselves. It may be one of the most misunderstood keys of transformation because most of our Wills are not free but encumbered with fear, blame, resentment, guilt, insecurity and shame from inappropriate and/or uninformed choices we have made, been encouraged to make, or been forced to make against our will.

The goal here is to free our Will by removing the factors and regiments of imprisonment of our Will to enable clear conscious choice by a Freed Will. Our actions are a result of thoughts, intentions, emotions and desire, and the Will actuates our actions. The important thing to take stock of is what is informing the Will. The Will is the voice of your essential deepest driving desires; your heart felt values and principles, your life purpose. If you are fluent in the language of your Soul (silence) and your Higher Self (intuition) and your Heart (emotions), your Will will be properly informed. If you do not hear or know those languages and you are only fluent in the language of your Mind (words), or your ego (thoughts), your Will may be confused, weakened or ill-advised and other intentions will win out. This is how the human Will has suffered criticism for some time. The problem is that inappropriate and harmful action is coming from some other intention and the Will has no power or is weakened in that moment. If we are committed to Pure Consciousness expressing through us, then our Will is the same as God's Will, powerful, discerning and strong. We are not our will.

8 - DESIRE - The Language of the Soul

In the silence of nature, solitude, meditation and/or prayer, with a silent mind, we can experience and hear our Soul. Our deepest driving desires, the key to our being and our reason for being. We live in a world where silence is at a premium. Much can be gained by arranging priorities so you can have those sacred moments of silence often. Your schedule doesn't matter, your responsibilities don't matter. What needs to be done is to access tranquility and strengthen the mind. The silence is really the ability to be calm in chaos. Being in nature, solitude, meditation and/or prayer and similar practices simply gives us the experience of that silence and your field responds with that experience. When you know yourself at the level of the Soul, where you live and why you are here, the silence is there and the pure desires of your being can be heard.

9 - CONSCIOUSNESS /Universal Mind/Unified Field - The Language of The Source of All Things

Meditation, ceremony and ritual and many healing practices can take us out of our normal perception of "reality" called Maya...the illusion. And those traditions are still a mainstay of spiritual evolution, for we cannot think our way into understanding consciousness. We live in uncommon times, and the illusion has become our reality more than ever with less time and contact with nature, silence or contemplation. Energy and information available to us within that illusion is massive and relentless and seems to support the truth of the illusion, and in a way, the technological environment is doing our thinking for us.

We have actually shifted the way we think and the search engines thinks for us. One benefit of that is the digital technology model gives us a better approximation of who we really are. The concept that everything is accessible energy and information is easy to understand now. Consciousness is the World Wide Web, the structure of the Universe, and we are exquisite search engines. When we begin to understand the true nature of the Universe and that is our true nature as well, we begin to be able to understand we are consciousness.

In my childhood and my early years of teaching, this was one of our biggest challenges. To communicate one had to be in person or "connected" by wires, and to access information, it had to be written or recorded, or received live from a person. The concept of being connected to all that was overwhelming.

The ancient texts describe an energy and information universe of pure consciousness and the ability to access it through intuited information and observation of nature. Not so recently, consciousness was a source of skepticism by many scientists, but current psychological and neurological scientific findings demonstrate that consciousness has a correlation with the ability to be present in the moment. It has also been shown that there are neural and psychological correlates to certain states of consciousness such as subliminal perception, phantom pain, denial of physical limitation, altered states. Consciousness indeed appears to be the primary source of all things, energy, light, pure potentiality, limitlessness, and unboundedness. The experience of these states through experience and healing practices, leads to expanded and pure awareness states of being, consciousness, and our true nature.

We are consciousness. Big belief gap!

...breathe...

Seven Everyday Vehicles of Transformation

1 – HIGHER STATES OF BEING - Your Luxury Vehicle

What you do speaks so loudly, I can't hear what you are saying.

-Ralph Waldo Emerson

Remember these are not concepts, ideas or actions...they are embodied, felt states of being. They are higher states of being because they involve "two-way love" and carry a high frequency vibration.

1. Gratitude – state of acknowledgement of all.

    Gratitude, Forgiveness and Compassion are not thoughts, ideas, concepts or actions. Each is felt states of being that has a specific effect on us and all others and all things, and are symptoms of enlightenment. They are all grounding and centering and change the environment for communication and relationship. Gratitude is an acknowledgement of all that we have including that which we do not want to have. It is the acknowledgement of the reality that currently surrounds us.

101

The state of gratitude is the highest frequency vibration in terms of the complete flow of energy/giving and receiving. In gratitude, we can assess, express and be content with what is. Otherwise, we are in the past or future or unaware. That is an imperative skill for living in the eternal now moment, the only real time we have.

NowOpp@Gratitude

To get a sense of the state of gratitude, get a pencil and paper and list twenty things you are grateful for, including the things you would just as soon not have. Next, using your non-dominant hand, list ten more things.

---

2. Forgiveness - state of kind knowing and forgiving.

Again, this is not a thought, idea, concept or action. It is not something we do because we think it's the right thing to do or that we have to do it. Forgiveness is an understanding that we are all doing the very best we can. Thoughtless, cruel, aggressive or covert actions towards us or others originate from unmet needs, and unconscious thinking. That includes actions that we originate towards others and towards ourselves, and self-forgiveness as well as forgiving others is a master key to personal and societal freedom. If we choose not to attempt forgiveness, we are perpetrating the cycle of abuse.

The reason it is so hard to forgive is because it is an energetic dynamic and thinking kind or forgiving thoughts will not work. Energy healing is truly effective in achieving forgiveness. It clears the triggers and trauma that hold regret, revenge and hatred in place.

3. Compassion - state of true understanding.

Because Compassion is not a thought, idea, concept or action, but a state of being, the way to be compassionate is to be compassion. It is a state of deep, unbiased, nonjudgmental empathy for whatever is in front of you. This state of being comes with practice and eventually becomes your normal state of being; it will influence all your thoughts and deeds, expand your conscious awareness and will afford joy, harmony and tranquility. Now that's a good investment in your Soul.

4. Awareness - state of full, clear acceptance.

Awareness could be called Grace. It is an opening of our perception, which is in turn an opening in our understanding and our ability to expand our consciousness. Awareness is the "ah-ha moment," the light bulb experience, the coincidence or synchronicity that gets our attention. It is something that triggers your curiosity, inner-knowing, compassion and forgiveness. It is a gift and sometimes a plea from the spirit to listen to the deeper meaning of whatever is going on. It can come in chaos but usually happens in a silent moment or a flower unfolding before your eyes. It is unmistakable when you are in grateful state of being.

The problem is, we have come to think that awareness is knowing the latest and greatest smart phone, pad or television show, political debate, business trend, fashion trend, fitness trend, workplace awareness, gossip, money-making opportunity, movie star or how to talk Starbuckese confidently. This is a sort of society survival awareness and leaves little room for Grace.

5. Humility – state of calm respect and willingness.

Humility is a state of tranquility fed by the knowingness that all things are transient. It has a present moment quality and a quality of great awareness. To be humble, one must be fully centered and grounded in one's beingness and still consciously aware of being connected to all things. It's difficult to tell a humble person, "I told you so!" Humility is a counter point to debilitating greed and pride.

6. Consciousness – The flow of universal intent.

Consciousness is usually qualified as an individual subjective awareness of an external factor or an internal factor in terms of thinking, attitudes, beliefs, knowledge and being conscious, awake, and aware. The collective consciousness is common awareness of groups with shared beliefs, ideas and moral attitudes which create a reality of its own.

In terms of holistic energy healing, cosmic consciousness is the pure potential evolutionary force that expresses through us expanding and creating higher understanding and awareness as a higher state of being leading to enlightenment or pure being. It is the primary source of all things and a vibratory level we can access for immediate manifestation, deep meditation, and the experience of timelessness, guidance, bliss and akin to our true nature.

The goal here is to allow cosmic consciousness to express fully through us and embody us. The methods, practices, therapies, techniques and technologies offered in the book all contribute to that goal.

2 - BREATHING - Sharing the Life Force Consciously

Deep Breathing is more important than all the vegetables you could possibly eat.

-Yogi Bhajan, Ph.D.

There is a breath pattern for every state of being. When we are tense or afraid, we either breathe in a shallow and fast manner or hold our breath. Our nervous system gets the signal and our body prepares for danger. This is the classic stress response. If we are relaxed and feeling safe and nurtured, we breathe in a deep manner and slowly with long deep breaths. The perfect reflection of this is either a sleeping baby or pet.

The reason the breath/Prana is a key to enlightenment is if we do not like our state of being, we can consciously change our breathing pattern to consciously change our state of being. Also, we can consciously practice particular kinds of breathing to obtain particular states of being. This conscious use of the breath is called Pranayam. This healing practice spans centuries and cultures and we will discuss it in detail in the extraordinary healing systems section of this book.

Strange that we are discussing how to breathe when we wouldn't be here if we didn't...since it is the function that punctuates our lives at birth and at death...since it is something we do 20 to 30,000 times a day, depending on how you breath and your activity level! So, I think you will agree that you could benefit from learning all you can about more conscious breathing. The intention here is to offer knowledge and experience to help you improve the quality of your breathing and therefore the quality of your life.

(Caution please: There are breathing exercises in this section and in the section on Pranayam. These exercises can cause dizziness. Please never force or overdo when doing breathing exercises. Thank you.)

NowOpp@YourBaseBreathRate

Get a timer or watch that has a second hand. Just breathe normally and count inhales for 60 seconds. Now multiply that number by 60 (minutes) and the total by 24 (hours) and that is approximately how many breaths you take a day.

What was true for me and what I have found is true for many is that we know very little about our bodies in actuality unless you are in the medical field, have had a lot of contact with anatomical studies, or a body worker of some kind. So, I would like to start with the actual mechanics of breathing.

It's embarrassing to admit that I made it all the way through 18 years of school and I didn't realize the lungs were simple sacs and depended on the movement of the thoracic muscles and diaphragms to inflate and deflate. When I began my holistic studies, I was surprised to learn the features and muscles of the head, face, ribs back and abdomen that are responsible for breathing along with many other factors.

NowOpp@HowYouBreathe

Experiment to get a sense of all that is going on. Place fingers between ribs and breathe in front and back...on sides...on collar bone...top of shoulders....palms over the eyes...over the ears... flare the nostrils...yawn....sigh...cough. Sit slouched over and try to breathe...now try to talk about something you are excited about... Now sit up, chest erect, shoulder down and talk and breathe.

The Four Components of a Complete Breath

Another thing I was unaware of were the four components of a complete breath:

- Inhale
- Pause
- Exhale
- Pause

NowOpp@FourPhasesOfBreath

Breathe the four phases in equal parts to the count of four:

Inhale 1,2,3,4 Pause 1,2,3,4 Exhale 1,2,3,4 Pause 1,2,3,4

Repeat two more times. You may notice a sense of relaxation.

This is actually the basis for a breathing practice/pranayam that stimulates the parasympathetic nervous system and the relaxation response. It is called the complete breath you can practice in increments of time up to 15 second segments, and is then called the one minute breath. That is a very advanced practice and should be very slowly approached over time. Never force the breath past comfort for the body.

The Four Stages of Breathing

Understanding complete respiration physiologically and metaphysically is a breakthrough step to awareness, and understanding of how prana/the life force moves through us, informs us and heals and balances us.

a. external respiration...air outside us taken into lungs
b. internal respiration...air from lungs to the blood
c. cellular respiration...from the blood to the cells
d. pranic respiration...into the subtle body within and outside the physical body

NowOpp@SecondAwarenessBreathingExercise

Keep reading and stay aware of your breathing.

Look around the room and count the white objects and remain conscious of your breathing.

Think of your to-do list and remain conscious of your breathing.

Get up and walk around, hum and remain conscious of your breathing.

This practice will raise your conscious awareness.

NowOpp@YourBaseBreathRate

Let's measure your base rate of breathing once again. Get a timer or watch that has a second hand. Just breathe normally and count inhales for 60 seconds.

More than likely, unless you already had a very low rate per minute, your rate has decreased from what it was at the first of the chapter and that is desirable. The breath is our most powerful and accessible healing tool, brings quick predictable results, and Pranayam should be a part of our every day.

3 - THINKING - Using the Minds Consciously

I did not arrive at my understanding of the fundamental laws of the Universe through my rational mind.

-Albert Einstein

Premises of Thinking, Believing and Creating Your Reality

- Everything is energy, vibration and information including thoughts, beliefs, images and physically-manifested things and situations.

- By raising our awareness of the vibratory quality of our thinking, we can shift negative or destructive thinking patterns and limiting beliefs.

- Conditioned, habitual, imbalanced and stressful thinking covers or clouds feelings/sensations/emotions.

- We are not our thoughts; we can't change thinking by thinking about it; feeling and our higher selves must be involved in changing negative thought patterns.

- Conscious use of the imagination/visualization is necessary for sustainable transformation/manifestation.

- Suppressed or conscious or unconscious thoughts and limiting beliefs manifest disconnect, negativity and destructive tendencies.

- Understanding the mind and its real makeup and function is the first step towards freedom or the nightmare of recurring destructive patterns and manifesting the life you really want.

- Through the practice of yoga, meditation and energy therapy, we can shift the processing of pure information through the proper channels and benefit from clearer, truer, healthier thinking and beliefs.

- The Will must be freed and strengthened to assure the elimination of old destructive patterns. The practice of non-judgment is the first step to freeing the Will.

- The images, emotions and meanings of situations and things are the basic units of human learning patterns and the rational mind/left brain function is not able to solve disrupted learning patterns. We must incorporate our creative mind/right brain function.

The Problem with 60,000 Thoughts a Day

It is estimated that we have 60,000 or more thoughts a day. The problem with that is most of them are the same thoughts we had yesterday, thinking things we already know. We want to be in a familiar comfort zone of energy and information and create safe reliable patterns. The problem is that some of those patterns are no longer applicable to our life or attached to some emotional turmoil. Soon we realize we are having the same thoughts over and over and become preoccupied about that and can't figure out how to get out of it. Lack of awareness of the dynamics of thinking, self-referral and questioning the self, contribute to circular thinking and obsessive thoughts and actions.

Thinking can be the wrecker or the corrector. The problem with thinking is over thinking and thinking the same thing over and over. The answer to the problem is understanding the brain and how it works and the fact that we have three minds, not one, and, simplistically, each mind has a specific talent and language. Using the rational mind to solve issues of the Heart doesn't work. And using the creative mind to make a list and carry out a task or do a math problem doesn't really work. Also, ignoring and bypassing the neutral mind and overriding with the rational mind are what debilitating stress is about. The goal here is to understand the basic functions of the brain, how to access all three of your minds and synchronize your brain with your heart.

Our brains will even "make things up" or adapt what is to make sense of something and fit it into our perceived reality. A good example is the following paragraph. If you can read it, you have a strong mind.

7H15 M3554G3 53RV35 70 PROVE3 H0W 0UR MIND5
C4N DO 4M4ZING 7HING5! 1MPR3551V3 7HING5!
1N 7HE B3GINN1NG 17 WA5 H4RD BU7 N0W, 0N 7H15
LIN3 Y0UR M1ND 1S R34D1NG 4B0U7 17, B3 PROUD!

The adaptive subconscious helps us make sense of things, however, if it is constantly adapting to past knowledge and isn't balanced with neutral (meditative thought) and creative (out of the box) thinking, or doesn't have enough time because of relentless stress, we can end up in the proverbial rut, or worse – making regretful decisions. The Will is more than likely left out of this cycle and it takes a toll on us physically and emotionally and spiritually, and our self-respect and self-confidence decline.

So, how do we think what we don't know? Think what you've never thought before? Not think only what someone else has thought or others think and possibly never have an original thought? It takes lateral, or out of the box thinking. Moving into the neutral and creative minds to balance the rational mind activity takes letting go of bias, control, and fear to open to new ideas. The first step is to be aware of your habitual thinking and underlying belief patterns.

To Recognize It Is To Transform It

Raise your consciousness to recognize and identify imbalanced thinking and transform it. This literally transforms your life. This allows the truth to surface which changes feelings and heightens the ability to manage our interactions and emotions. The quality of your life will soar.

Please put your attention on the lists below of examples of limiting belief thinking and expanding belief thinking and constructive thinking and distorted thinking. Assess your own thinking. Which lists are more predominant in your own thinking patterns? Make a conscious practice of becoming aware of the difference when you hear yourself speaking, and move into the belief patterns and constructive thinking of the B lists and to observe the shifts in your sense of being.

What Are Your Basic Thought Motivations That Lead to Your Actions?

A List - Competitive:
1. I have to accomplish a lot to feel good.
2. I'm in it to win.
3. I need to hurry.
4. There is not enough time.
5. I should know.
6. I need approval.
7. I need to be the best.
8. I need to wear and use a watch frequently.
9. I need to constantly improve and achieve.
10. I can and should do it all.

B List – Contributive:
1. Just a sense of being feels good.
2. I'm in it to learn and experience.
3. Time expands to meet my needs.
4. All in good time.
5. I can know.
6. Acceptance of myself brings me peace.
7. Cooperative efforts nurtures greatness.
8. I instinctively know what time it is.
9. I am a work in progress.
10. It is not all for me to do.

A List - Too Positive or Too Negative

1. All or Nothing Thinking – characterized with words like always/never black/white.
2. Overgeneralization – the belief that a bad apple spoils all the other apples.
3. Mental Filter – the belief that one drop of ink in a gallon of water changes the meaning of the water.
4. Disqualifying the Positive - positive as random, rare, and negative as the ordinary and inevitable.
5. Jumping to Conclusions – from one fact, idea or statement, assuming you know all facts, also called mind reading and future telling.
6. Magnification or Making the Ordinary a Catastrophe - minimizing or exaggerating to justify or embellish yourself or your story.
7. Emotional Reasoning - I feel it is true, therefore it is true (this is not intuition).
8. Should Statements - must, should, ought to, got to statements are driven by guilt/fear and generate fear and guilt.
9. Labeling/Mislabeling - labeling yourself or others is judgment personified.
10. Personalization – characterizing someone in relation to your opinion of yourself - superior, inferior, self-importance, defensive.
11. Deal Thinking – if I do this then, that will happen – gambling with relationship.

B List – Balanced Protective/Projective/Neutral/Healing

1. Solution Possibility Thinking - creative, original, considerate.
2. Discerning Difference - feeling each essence.
3. Seeing the Whole Picture - clear authentic assessment.
4. Balancing with Positive - recognizing and gratitude.
5. Using the Neutral Mind – compassionate communication, balance, honesty, integrity.
6. Neutral Mind/Heart - determine source of emotions.
7. Balanced Mind/Heart - determine right action.
8. Balanced Positive Mind/Heart - determine real message.
9. Neutral Mind - determine situation dynamics and balance.
10. No Deals – conscious choice.

Thoughts and Emotions – The Debate

One ought to hold on to the heart; for if one lets it go, one soon loses control of the head too.

-Friedrich Nietzsche

Many behavioral psychologists feel that thoughts create emotions. I used to subscribe to the belief that emotions cause thoughts. We would have great debates about it to no real agreement. Now, I believe that both theories are correct.

What brought me to that conclusion was the study of the mind during my Kundalini teacher certification process and particularly studying the book, *The Mind, Its projections and Multiple Facets*, by Yogi Bhajan, Ph.D., who was responsible for bringing Kundalini Yoga to the western hemisphere in the sixties. The book is based on universal laws and holistic principles. All is one, nothing is separate and there is no beginning or end. That every thought, word and deed has an effect and consequence for the whole.

The two charts below from *The Mind*, explain that thoughts, emotions, desires and actions are all part of one cycle. They are all energetic components of the mind/body function. There is really no cause and effect and the outcome depends upon what influences are or are not applied during the cycle of intellect, thought, emotion, desire and action. The charts also take into consideration the universal mind/unified field, the interaction of facets/words, and beliefs of the rational mind, thoughts, the language of the ego, emotion, the language of the heart, desire, the language of the soul and action, the language of the Will.

The whole cycle of thought is a process of our entire existence. The problems come, in my opinion, with our former lack of awareness of the wholeness and interrelatedness of the thinking cycle and putting our attention on only one aspect of the cycle such as thoughts, emotions, desires or actions, and in most cases, in my experience, ignoring the power and purpose of the Will. The phrase, *broaden your thinking*, takes on new meaning in this light.

By speaking the languages of you fluently, it is possible to intercede at any point on the chart of the dynamic process of whole thinking, to undo the reasons you sometimes create desires and actions that are detrimental or destructive. Many people complain that "...they are doing so well and then fall off the wagon again..." These are some of the best known pitfalls of a faulty or undesirable thought cycle consequence:

- Lack of awareness of the part the universal mind/unified field plays in your thinking cycle
- A-List thinking patterns
- Lack of a regular spiritual healing practice to calm the mind and emotions and know the universal mind/unified field
- Not knowing your principles and beliefs
- Letting things go that bother you and allowing emotions to take over
- Not engaging the creative mind for images of a desired consequence
- Lack of fluency and trust in the languages of you or silencing them with drugs, alcohol, too much stress, etc.
- Denying your Will in favor of pleasing others

Self assessment and learning and awareness and acknowledgment of thinking patterns are enough to turn the tide of destructive thinking. Take time to evaluate your own thinking. Include your creative mind and emotions as guides in the evaluation. From here, attention on opportunities to self-reflect on the process as you go through it, will help you understand the dynamic and skillfully work through it. Learning and doing holistic practices and energy healing methods will enable you to go through the cycle with expanded awareness and grace and ease.

The Dynamic Process of Whole Thinking -
Choice Points of Influence

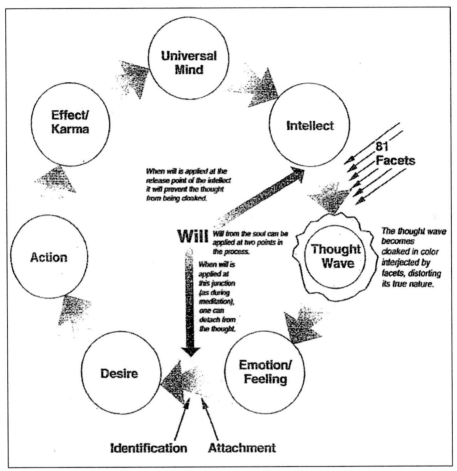

Chart from *The Mind, Its Projections and Multiple Facets*, by Yogi Bhajan, PhD

Insights and Guidance for Better Thinking Paths

Three Functional Minds	Aspects Functional Minds X Impersonal Minds	Controlling Projections Aspect Interacting With Functional Mind	Guiding Phrase
Negative Mind	Negative Mind X Manas/senses/ Defender	Negative-Soldier Positive-Ombudsman Neutral-Prospector	How to deal with a threat How to deal with an accident How to deal with a coincidence
Negative Mind	Negative Mind X Ahangkar/Ego/ Manager	Negative-Historian Positive-Chameleon Neutral-Judge	Relay of a past memory Phrase of a mental projection Shadow of a mental projection
Negative Mind	Negative Mind X Buddhi/seeks truth /Preserver	Negative-Runner Positive-Integrator Neutral-Apostle	Deep memory of a past projection Mental intersection Mental outer projection
Positive Mind	Positive Mind X Manas/senses/Artist	Negative-Actor Positive-Architect Neutral-Entrepreneur	The art of memorizing creativity The art of creating art The art of creating creativity
Positive Mind	Positive Mind X Ahanghar/Ego/ Producer	Negative-Gourmet Positive-Architect Neutral-Creator	Creating art through past memory Creating art by environmental effects Creating art by projecting into the future
Positive Mind	Positive Mind X Buddhi/Seeks Truth/Missionary	Negative-Devotee Positive-Enthusiast Neutral-Creator	Pursuing the cycle of success Pursuing the cycle of artistic attributes Pursuing the art of cohesiveness
Neutral Mind	Neutral Mind X Manas/Senses/ Strategist	Negative-Scout Positive-Coach Neutral-Guide	Judging environments through senses Judging environments Judging positive environments through intuition
Neutral Mind	Neutral Mind X Ahangkar/Ego/ Leader	Negative-Protector Positive-Commander Neutral-Pathfinder	Assessment of position Assessment of the successful Assessment of personality & facets through intuition
Neutral Mind	Neutral Mind X Buddi/Seeks Truth/ Teacher	Negative-Educator Positive-Expert Neutral-Master	Intuitive assessment of personality defects to be covered Interpretations of all facets of life Assessment of personality overloads and their projections to be controlled

Chart from *The Mind, Its Projections and Multiple Facets*, by Yogi Bhajan, PhD

115

A Word about the Brain Itself

We can thank the neuroscientists, metaphysicists, researchers and visionary medical and healing professionals and organizations for evolving our thinking about our brains exponentially. As you may recall, it was not too long ago that we thought that in terms of brain power and brain function, was "what you got is all you have, so do your best with what you got." The whole nuture/nature debate about the influence of the nature of a persona versus environmental influences on growth and development still goes on.

The holistic approach considers all influences and limitless possibilities of discovery and awareness allowing us to recover our innate wisdom and abilities. Thankfully, healing systems are merging now and resulting in huge advancements in understanding and healing of the brain. We know that nutrition and how we choose to use our brains directly affect how our brains function. We are now aware of the devastation caused by drugs and alcohol, compulsive bad habits, television, cell phones and relentless stress on the brain's health and function. Remember, how you use and treat your brain determines how your brain functions.

It is an exciting time and unfolding quickly. I urge you to learn as much as you can about your brain. Below is a list of resources of some of the work in this field of brain health I have found visionary and game changing.

Thinking Resource Guide

Super Brain by Deepak Chopra, M.D. & Rudolf E. Tanzi, Ph.D.
Change Your Brain, Change Your Life, By Daniel Amen
Molecules of Emotion, by Candace Pert, Ph.D.
My Stroke of Insight, by Jill Bolte Tayor, Ph.D.
Power vs. Force, by David R Hawkins, M.D., Ph.D.
The Mind, Its projections and Multiple Facets, By Yogi Bhajan Ph.D.
The Brain That Changes Itself, by Norman Doidge
Blink, The Power of Thinking Without Thinking, by Malcolm Gladwell
Biology of Belief, by Bruce Lipton, Ph.D.
Energy Medicine, by Donna Eden
Esoteric Anatomy, by Bruce Burger
Soul Connection CD, Guided Meditations and Energy Healing, by Andrea Becky Hanson

The Power of Mental Imaging

How have you learned what you know? Who, what and where has influenced you and taught you what you know? How do you remember what you have learned? Why do you remember seemingly unrelated, random, incidents from long ago? What makes you remember them? What makes something stick in your memory? How are you learning what you don't know yet?

The reason it is important to understand the dynamics of learning is so you can "unlearn" correct or transform detrimental perceptions and beliefs, and raise your conscious awareness of incoming information.

There is so much research about learning, brain function and memory, it is mind boggling! There is one area I am particularly interested in sharing with you because it explains a powerful tool of healing and transformation which is the power of an image. A picture is truly worth a 1,000 words and an image is worth infinite amounts of information.

A very interesting study shows that the average child recognizes over 200 company logos by the time he/she enters first grade. Most children will recognize more logos than letters in the alphabet by the time they are three. Learning logos is part of environment imprinting and works by association. The child sees the logo/sign and associates it with the next activity or experience which gives the sign meaning. McDonald's for example means food. It can also mean, "Fun" or "where I get a toy" or "where I get what I want" or "where I never get what I want." Smell, touch, sounds and tastes associated with environmental imprinting images can also conjure up the associated meanings and feelings attached to the image.

The visionary psychologist, Akhter Ahsen, Ph.D., author of over 30 books, pioneered psychotherapy based in mental imagery, an innovative field in modern psychology in the early 1950's called, Eidetic Therapy. What he found is that images actually carried two other components: the somatic emotion or body sensation, and the meaning contained in the visual experience. He discovered and developed the I (Image) S (Somatic/Feeling) M (Meaning/Belief) Model – the basic human learning unit. This was monumental because it identified the possible intervention of triggers that can block the growth and natural talents and expression of an individual. This is a continuous process and looks like this:

I S M I S M I S M I S M I S M I S M I S M I
S M I S M I S M I S M I S M I S M I S M I S M
I S M I S M I S M I S M I S M I S M I S
M I S M I S M I S M I S M I S M I S M I
S M I S M I S M I S M I S M I S

Using Eidetic Therapy, the associations are changed and corrected through specific mental imaging, which causes a change in the brain's associations and consequently releases the triggers of negative associations.

With the use of Energy Therapies, we track the origin of the triggers, using talk therapy and energy testing and tapping to dislodge the energy interruptions in the energy body, which results in a different perception (ISM unit) of the problem. We can also use mental imaging, visualization and creative visualization to change the image and that results in a change in the outcome. So to change the undesired reality...change the image.

When I was first learning these methods, I applied it to an "unexplainable" overreaction I found myself repeating. I will share the whole realization and outcome with you. As a sixth grader, I had experienced the very tragic image of my dear devoted dog, Pete, a slick-haired white terrier with a black eye, getting hit by a truck. I ran into the street and picked him up and he died in my arms. I was devastated as you can imagine. I didn't have another dog for a long, long time. Until about ten years later after I was married and we decided to get a dog. We chose a St. Bernard. I was very protective of her and wouldn't let her go anywhere near traffic. It was the same with our second and third Saints. It was easy, because they don't tend to run away. Then we got two St. Bernards and one of them, Sierra, was a runner....she thought she was a lab. We lived in a rural area and she and my daughter's dog, Doggie, a slick-haired terrier/pit bull with a black eye, would run off and I noticed I would get inappropriately scared and be yelling and screaming at them to come back. I tried every kind of training professional and long leashes to train them not

118

to run away to no avail. And in the meantime, I was embarrassed about how outrageously upset I would get when they would run off. It was during this time I was learning about the power of imagery and Eidetic Therapy procedures. One day when I saw Sierra and Doggie dig under the gate to get out, I had an epiphany...I had never had the thought that Doggie looked just like Pete. The whole incident came back to my consciousness and I felt the sadness and horror all over again. At that moment, I realized why I was inappropriately reactive when they ran away...my subconscious image was that they would be killed. So I applied what I had learned about changing the image, and associated fear and sadness and the belief that when my dog runs away, he gets killed. I consciously imagined that when I called them they would stop, turn around and come back. It took several attempts over three or four days for me to disarm the old image, feel authentic with the new image, and for them to figure out the new commands, but it worked!

As adults, we have literally millions of environment imprints, conscious and subconscious images with which we associate feelings/emotions and meaning/thoughts and beliefs. Some bring joy and fulfillment resulting in healthy well-being, and some bring sorrow or negative memories and can be debilitating and produce traumatic stress, anxiety, depression and the like, resulting in emotional turmoil and repeated stress and even poor health. Holistic energy healing is the key to resolving and correcting the debilitating imprints and related emotions. I am continually thankful that my life path has brought me to this position of teaching and writing about this fabulous good news and spreading the word.

Conscious Beliefs and Principles

Our beliefs create our reality, what do you believe?

-Andrea Becky

- Your beliefs create your reality and your consequent thoughts, actions and desires.
- Being conscious of your beliefs brings consciousness to your thoughts and actions.

- Do you know yours? Take time to feel them and write them down. They shape your life... best to know.
- These are mine that I developed and wrote in my journal dated 9/19/99. They have served me well, and I am happy to share them.

I believe that I only need begin where I am
that now is where I begin and end
that eternity exists in each moment
that I create my reality with each choice
that the past can be changed with each thought and action

I believe that all is one
that understanding replaces judgment
that we can heal only ourselves
that all healing occurs from within
that the highest good is balance

I believe my purpose is to fully love and accept myself and others
to remember and express honestly, authentically and freely
to be centered in kindness
to listen to my heart and live in gratitude
to know and use my unique talents
and to share what I discover along the way
Andrea revised 2001

Belief Resource Guide:

Psycheye, by Akhter Ahsen, M.D.
Reinventing the Body, Resurrecting the Soul, by Deepak Chopra, M.D.
Biology of Belief, by Bruce H. Lipton, Ph.D.
Blink - The Power of Thinking Without Thinking, by Malcolm Gladwell

4 - MEDITATING - Using Consciousness Consciously

Meditation 101 - A Broad Base of Information about Meditation

Meditation is a great adventure inward. The ultimate discovery of your own unbounded personal power and the ability to access it at will. It is an adventure into what we have forgotten or what has been lost from our awareness. It is a path to understanding our true unique and universal and multidimensional nature. It is a practice that changes your state of being, perception, and expands awareness and consciousness. It is called "a practice" because it is a practice of accessing your true identity, your essential self, your natural state of perfect health, serenity, knowingness, gratitude and love. It is a process of experiencing all aspects of ourselves and all that is around us in clearer and deeper ways.

Basically, it is putting your attention on something in a certain way with a particular intention.

From the beginning of time, most cultures have used forms of meditation as part of their daily routine. Each culture and subculture has developed representative forms of meditation using sound and silence, movement and stillness, music and rhythm; some with roots in prayer and as prayer, some as celebration of significant passages, some as introspection and self-realization, and some as transcendence. There are hundreds of ways to meditate from silent and still, to loud with radical movement and everything in between. All meditation forms have evolved out of the human desire for deeper understanding, meaning, knowing and connection to the divine, to self, to others and to the universe, and are seen as the path to enlightenment.

What Meditation Is Not

For eons, meditation has existed in many different forms and many different cultures. In the western world, meditation had received only mild acceptance. I feel this is because of the confusion about what meditation really is. Meditation is not a dogma, religion, hypnosis or magic, although the results of meditation often feel magical. Our western nation's high industrialization and importance put on academic and scientific approaches to understanding and learning seemed to exclude meditation as a viable integrative option for learning and understanding.

Paradoxically, now it is the scientific community, specifically quantum physicists, neuroscientists and neuroanatomists and progressive members of the medical and research professions, which has been responsible for a great surge in interest in and practice of meditation. Their latest findings about actual makeup of the human and the universe collaborate with those of the ancient seers. We are the benefactors of the two paths meeting around the understanding of the true nature of the human and of the universe. We know now that scientifically or spiritually that we are not alone. No matter what path you take, there is definitely more to us than meets the eye. And that "more than meets the eye" appears to be our essential state that is known to be accessible through regular meditation practice. Remember, meditation is not something you do, it is an evolutionary process. Also, my experience has been that what I began meditating for is now just a mile post along the way. The benefits and experiences have far surpassed anything I could have imagined.

Why Meditate?

The reasons for meditating range from desiring a deep and holy experience to wanting simple techniques for relaxation and better health. We know that it releases stress and balances the nervous system. It calms our minds and allows our body to heal. It increases our capacity for living and insight and understanding. The greatest benefit is it works on all levels, physical, mental, emotional, spiritual, and environmental and basically, it is effortless. It is a whole field experience of a level of our being not otherwise experience-able and brings fitness to all levels of our being. What will appeal to you and will work best for you will depend on your basic nature, beliefs and life patterns. But what remains is that meditation is a very basic transformational vehicle and I highly recommend developing a regular practice of some kind if you haven't already.

Everyone's experience of the transforming nature of meditation is different for individual reasons. I remember clearly my first experiences. Everything was brighter. I noticed flowers and beauty so accentuated that I believed it wasn't there before and would ask if it was new. The other gift was time and space. I was reactive by nature growing up and especially in confrontation since my defense mechanism of choice was anger. What I noticed after meditating regularly for a short time, was I felt like I had time to hear and see what was happening, assess what I saw and/or heard, and choose the course of action I felt was the most beneficial. It was a process instead of a reaction. And, the more I meditated, the more all of me wanted to meditate...including my very active mind. I believe that was from experiencing the timelessness of the field and the truth of my own true makeup of timelessness.

Fourteen Meditation Practice Keys – Look Familiar?

Notice that you already possess all these keys. Using your keys and integrating them with different kinds of meditations (listed below) can give you an idea of the vastness of meditation possibilities and experience.

- Perception – The Reality Creator
- Attention – The Life Giver
- Intention – Fuel of Manifestation
- Experience – The Memory Keeper
- Awareness – The Door Opener
- Breath – The Universal Life Force
- Sensation – The Awakener
- Emotion – The Informer
- Imagination – The Igniter
- Memory – The Reminder
- Movement – The Integrator
- Creativity – The Innovator
- Silence – Where the Truth is
- Reflection – The Reality Checker

A Meditation Sampler - Brief Descriptions and Examples of Various Meditation Techniques

There are as many meditation techniques as there are people meditating, however, there are general categories of meditation that have specific technique and intent that are good to be aware of. In the end, what will appeal to you will depend on your individual nature and the nature of your environment and what your desires and intentions are. Remember that nothing is separate, so any meditation, for any reason, will have an effect on you. Below are general categories of meditation and their brief descriptions. Your use and choice depend upon your needs, desires and interests.

- Breath Awareness – for health and fitness at all levels, focus on and alter the breath in prescribed ways. This is called Pranayam and is addressed at length in the Healing Practices part of the book.
- Chanting and Toning - for higher consciousness and integration of the body, mind, spirit and will for healing vibration from the inside out.
- Concentration – to exercise and balance the brain, concentrate on an object, any aspect of nature, candle light, mandala, with soft eyes, with your full attention on the aspects of the object.
- Contemplation – to develop and strengthen the neuropathways of the brain, contemplate possibilities of a concept, problem or situation.
- Creative Activity Meditations – gardening, cooking, artwork, sewing, writing or journaling, certain sports and hobbies that result in a sense of timelessness and relaxation.
- Creative Visualization - the power of visualization and sensation of desired conscious thoughts, images and outcomes created in your mind's eye.
- Cultural and Religious Meditations and Prayer – various ceremonies, rituals, prayers and meditations which are inherent with the cultural beliefs and practices. These often have to do with the rite of passage at certain ages, initiations, holidays, pre and post-event celebrations and ceremonial prayers.

- Guided Imaging – a facilitated, guided script to create specific images for a specific purpose. Commonly used in medical situations.
- Guided Visualization - a facilitated visualization with a specific intent scripted to create a certain outcome.
- Journaling as a Meditation Conscious Written Introspection
- Mantra, Sutra and Sound Meditation - repeating, mentally or vocally, basic sounds and/or words and phrases to integrate the finite with the infinite from the inside out. Also, using sounds of bells, tones, bowls, instruments such as the harp or gong, zither, drums, harmoniums, etc. to entrain (tune) the body, mind and spirit.
- Mental Imaging - to relax and increase body awareness and integrate body, mind and spirit and environment. Often used in medical de-stress and disease recovery programs.
- Mindful Meditation – the practice of being consciously aware of the breath, thoughts, ideas, beliefs, actions and deeds as a path to enlightenment.
- Moving Meditations- increasing flow of chi/prana, transcending and feeling and processing and integrating emotional energy. Includes Tai Chi, Qigong, Hatha Yoga.
- Self-Inquiry, Introspection - self-assessment, self-pledges, self-awareness.
- Yoga – a moving meditation for the purpose of integrating the infinite with the finite.
- Kundalini Yoga and Meditation – prescribed movement, chanting, breath patterns, mantra and sound music, teachings, spiritual and human evolution and integration of the finite and infinite.

Samples of Meditations Using Keys

> ### NowOpp@CreativeVisulization Meditation
> ### Imagination and Intention and Visualization
>
> - Be comfortable, take some deep breaths and relax and close your eyes.
> - Imagine something you want to happen and how you want it to happen.

- With clear and pure intention, begin to visualize in as detailed way as you can, what it is you want?
- When and where does this happen?
- Who else is there?
- Include yourself, colors, landscapes and environments.
- What does it look like, feel like, smell like, sound like?
- What emotions do you want to experience?
- What outcome do you want to experience?
- When you feel complete, be in gratitude for the experience and slowly open your eyes and transition to your next activity.

NowOpp@MindfulMeditation
Breath and Mindful Meditation

- Set a timer of some kind at five, ten, 15 or 20 minutes. Whatever you prefer.
- Sit comfortably, take one or two deep breaths, and relax.
- Allow your attention to go to your breathing. Simply observe your breath as it moves. Just witness it and do not try to change it.
- As you observe your breath, it may change. It may be faster, slower, deeper or shallower. It may even seem to stop. Just observe it.
- Your attention may drift away from your breath to something else. Simply bring your attention back to your breath.
- For the next few minutes try not to have any expectations you may have about this meditation and simply practice keeping your attention on your breath.
- Continue for the specified amount of time.
- At the end, take plenty of time when opening your eyes to transition to activity.

NowOpp@Biofieldcleansing
A Kundalini Yoga Moving Meditation

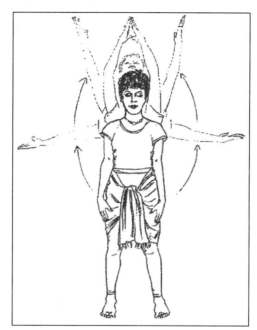

- Stand easily on the floor, feet shoulder-width apart with the eyes closed and rolled up to the third eye (middle of the forehead).
- Inhale very fully and deeply as your sweep your arms to the sky. Let your palms meet briefly overhead.
- Exhale powerfully as you sweep your arms down to the sides of your legs as if they were great wings.
- Flap them back up again, continuing the movement – inhaling as you reach to the heavens.
- Exhale as your bring your arms down to your sides.
- Time: one to three minutes.
- End: Sit or stand for a minute with your eyes closed, assess your aura, feeling its vastness.
- Effects: Doing this exercise will recharge the eighth chakra, your electromagnetic field and strengthen your blow. Do this exercise any time you are feeling disconnected, or a little dim. It is a very integrative movement, and it will help you to feel brighter and more whole almost immediately.

A Must-Use Self-Inquiry Meditation

There is one meditation that I feel we cannot do without. It can be done at anytime, anywhere, with the eyes open or closed, standing or seated or laying down and it can change your life and ability to access your inner goings on. I call it the Check-In-And-Ask Meditation. It involves simply directing your attention inward and checking in with yourself with self-inquiry. This is simple, fast, life-changing in the moment, and over time, helps with fluency in the languages of you. This technique also helps you become an expert at making great decisions in the now at choice point.

NowOpp@CheckInAndAskMeditation

Take a couple of deep breaths and now simply direct your attention within. Ask sincerely, in self-inquiry, "What's up?"... "How are you doing?" Just listen and feel what your field has to say. If everything is, okay, simply say, "Nice to connect, thank you." And be on your way. If everything is not okay, listen and do what is necessary to resolve the problem. This practice keeps you on track and aware of your needs and you will find you are a very interesting person!

Note: Meditation will be addressed again in Sections IV under Meditation and VI as part of Kundalini Yoga and Meditation.

Meditation Resource Guide:

Primordial Sound Meditation – www.chopra.com
Meditation as Medicine, Activate the Power of Your Natural Healing Force, by Dharma Singh Khalsa, M.D., and Cameron Stauth
Soul Connection, Guided Meditation and Energy Healing for Extraordinary Health and Well-Being, by Andea Becky Hanson
Meditation, The Complete Idiot's Guide, by Joan Budilovsky and Eve Adamson
Creative Visualization, Use the Power of Your Imagination to Create What You Want in Your Life, by Shakti Gawain

5 - EMOTIONAL FITNESS™ - A Foundation for Freedom and Joy

What is Emotional Fitness?

Emotional Fitness is a neutral state of being and dual awareness. The ability to travel through joy, sorrow, happiness, grief, love, hate, jealously, contentment, peace, chaos and more, and remain fully connected, balanced and aware of the greater and deeper meaning of life.

-Andrea Becky

The Emotional Fitness process has roots in an aspect of my Greek heritage, that of freely expressing, (perhaps to a fault) emotion and passion. It felt healthy to me and I liked knowing how people really felt and also being able to express how I felt too. I remember that I had the typical problems of a young girl growing up, and the typical emotions as well. I don't remember ever really getting taken down by the emotions of disappointment, or sadness, or anger.

My friends' families were quite different, and it seemed to me that emotional issues seemed to hang around and stack up for them at times. They became a sustained reality or part of their identity of sorts. It just felt uncomfortable and I never gave it much more thought than what I am explaining here and now. As I learned, I remained "solution-oriented" through rough times and depended on the security of structure and schedule.

With very few exceptions, this remained true for me for a long time. When I began owning my healing abilities and working with people that wanted help, I began to see the abundance of emotional turmoil and the inability to move through it on the part of my clients. It prompted me to begin developing my programs with emotional health and well-being as a focus. I began to realize that emotional turmoil was the leading obstacle to personal health and spiritual growth for most of my clients.

I started to use the Seven Step Emotional Release and Clearing process we developed at the Chopra Center. It was a very powerful and effective tool. It could be done with one person or several hundred and it was very well-received. Through teaching this process, I could see the full impact of most people's inability to process emotions in a healthy way and the relief from learning this process. It is mainly a cognitive process with encouraged creative methods for clearing.

NowOpp@EmotionalClearing
Seven Step Emotional Clearing

1. <u>Take Responsibility</u> for what you are feeling. It may be relative to another person, but they are more than likely some quality within you. If you take responsibility for your own feelings, you will not be as triggered and more able to resolve the feelings.
2. <u>Identify The Emotion</u> - Identify what it is you are feeling. Refer to the list of emotions in the appendices if you are having trouble identifying it. Describe it as well as you can and what is behind it, if possible.
3. <u>Witness the Sensation</u> in your body that represents the emotion. That is probably what brought your attention to the emotion. Just allow the feeling and let it move and express. This simple step will clear your field enough to hear the true message of the emotion.
4. <u>Express the Emotion to Yourself</u> by talking, writing, associating it with memories, thoughts and wishes and ideas you have about it.
5. <u>Release the Emotions</u> through some ritual like a fire ceremony, writing it down and burying it, physical movement, dancing, pranayam, vigorous exercise. Once, when I was asking for ideas about ways to express the emotions to yourself to a large group, a woman in the audience stood up and said, "I am going to call myself on my cell phone and rant and rage and then listen to it later." I thought that was brilliant.

---

6. <u>Share the Experience of the Emotion</u> - If you wish to and want to, share the experience and the feelings with a trusted friend without trying to solve the problem. If it is appropriate, share it with someone like a counselor or clergyman. Also, if it is appropriate, taking full responsibility for your feelings, you might share it with a person or persons involved in the situation that caused the emotions within you with the intent of resolution if necessary.
7. <u>Rejuvenate</u> by doing something pleasant for yourself like a massage, music, favorite food, walk in nature and nourish yourself.

In a way, not necessarily in this order, this is what happened around our home quite often. But it wasn't as conscious as this process.

Emotion – Energy in Motion

Every feeling is a field of energy. A pleasant feeling is an energy which can nourish. Irritation is a feeling which can destroy. Under the light of awareness, the energy of irritation can be transformed into an energy which nourishes.

-Thich Nhat Hahn

What I noticed about this seven-step process was it worked, people felt better, they could even see the humor in how upset they were, but most of the time, it didn't really get to the source of why the emotion was so intense and/or was even an issue. At the same time, I saw an incredible increase in the amount of people that were beginning to take medication for anxiety, depression and other emotional upset. I was also studying addiction and the reasons for addictive behavior and noticing that emotional turmoil more often than not preceded debilitating addictive habits and behaviors. The general public was spending billions of dollars "not to feel" on antidepressants, addictions of all sorts, like shopping, alcohol, drugs, sex, gambling...At the same time, I was beginning to study energy medicine and that was the missing piece to the puzzle of addiction and emotional turmoil.

The Nature of Emotional Energy

Asking the rational mind to resolve emotional problems is like vacuuming the family room with a lawn mower. It seems to work but causes a lot of damage.

-Andrea Becky 2013

All energy is endless and continuous and seeking dynamic balance through motion. Emotional Energy, as the language of the heart, our central synthesizer or our energy system, must be able to move, inform and keep moving for optimum emotional health and well-being. If the sensation of the emotional energy is suppressed, ignored, anesthetized or otherwise slowed or stopped, then not only is the message missed, but emotional turmoil ensues and our entire system is compromised.

In addition, when we are upset, we are usually happy if we can get to some kind of calm or resolved state, however, the likelihood of falling back into emotional turmoil is very high in that state. What is really needed is not only resolution and calm, but the next step which is rejuvenation and inspiration to keep the emotional energy moving and informing us of the things that nurture us like joy, peace and tranquility.

This realization is what prompted me to create the Emotional Fitness Healing Retreat concept. What I knew was that the negative emotional energy releasing process was absolutely necessary, and the supporting healing technologies were absolutely necessary to insure total success. The source of the triggers for negative emotion are found and cleared when the experience of the empowering technology was made available to each person. Also, the resulting strengthening of the nervous system and the elevation of the spirit are necessary to reach the realization of our true nature...one of peace, joy, and tranquility. This was a wonderful discovery journey.

Emotional Fitness Training is about the integration of knowledge, awareness and experience of the true nature of emotional energy (Energy Anatomy), the clearing of negative or debilitating thoughts and emotions (Energy Medicine), the resolution of the source of them (Energy Psychology), the technologies to strengthen the systems of the body, mind and spirit, and the ability to sustain Emotional Fitness

(Holistic Studies, Energy Psychology, Ayurveda, Kundalini Yoga and Meditation, Pranayam and Interdimensional Healing).

We cannot reach our goals or spiritual growth, heightened awareness and expanded consciousness without the ability to hear and interpret and act upon the languages of us, especially the language of our Heart, emotions.

Resource:

www.mergingrivers.com
www.facebook.com/MergingRiversHealingPractices

6 - MOVEMENT - Using the Body Consciously

Conscious movement of all kinds; stillness, silence, physical action, thinking thoughts, speaking words, following beliefs, devotional acts, feeling emotions, put you in sync with nature. Practicing the integrity of conscious awareness of movement of all kinds leads to enlightenment.

-Andrea Becky

You Were Made to Move – Holistic Fitness

Moving the body with conscious intent and focus changes and adjusts your relationship with your body as well as your energy field which are the fields of truth. Since the body is the ultimate measurer of the presence of truth, it is necessary to develop a more intimate and compassionate relationship with it for optimum health and well-being.

Physical movement, particularly yoga, dancing, and bilateral movements, stimulates the power centers of the body (chakras), causes movement through the energy channels (meridians), and cleanses and balances the whole field (biofield). Conscious intentional movement of the physical body stimulates the creative integrating power centers of the field...the imaginative mind, the Will and the Heart center. To transcend mental conditioning and "stuckness" on any level, physical, mental, emotional or spiritual, movement is the key. Using physical movement in a conscious way to emphasize and express thoughts and emotions helps getting unstuck and become more balanced. The solution for artists, writers and all creative endeavors in which we sometime feel stuck, is movement.

Movement accompanied by music offers increased benefits. Sound causes movement vibrationally, as well. If it is a pleasant rhythm and beat, melody, lyrics, etc., it increases the healing effect because the body, mind and spirit entrain/sympathize with the harmony and rhythm. This goes for music from the inside out too, like singing, humming, whistling and chanting.

About Yoga – The Adventure in Consciousness

Yoga's origins are in the human experience and are thousands of years old. Its techniques are all about leading a happy, healthy, spiritually aware life. Although yoga is sometimes thought of as mystical, it is steeped in the human sciences and based on observations of energy and the effects of different activities on the individual energy. Yogic activities include body positions, called *asanas*; hand and eye position, called *mudras*; motion of the breath, called *pranayam*; instruments of the mind, called *mantras/ meditation*, music and *chanting*; and the flow of consciousness, called the *naad*. Yoga means union, yoke, unite or experiencing *two energies*, specifically, the finite and the infinite, together and into balance. The wisdom offered by yoga depends on your own practice and discipline. Yoga is a practice in the experience of the merging of the finite and the infinite.

Aspects of Yoga

Yoga is a vast human science with twenty-two forms of yoga based on specific disciplines and intent and hundreds of kinds of branches of those main forms. Patanjali, the ancient seer, envisioned 195 sutras/ thought provoking aphorisms that remain a definitive foundation of yoga. They are based on the premise that knowledge is awakening and even redeeming and it is through clarity, intuition, and understanding the timeless nature of the Self, that we can transcend suffering

134

and stop the unconscious thinking, beliefs and actions that create problems. I am offering here just a taste of the comprehensive and multilayered nature of yoga for your consideration and awareness and study. Please note references at the end of this section for more detail ,if you wish.

The six schools of yogic philosophies and emphasis:

1. Purva-Mimamsa/individual responsibility for one's actions and free will to create quality of life
2. Vedanta/internal experience and the nature of meditation, the mystic scriptures and integrated right action with the Oneness of creation and the nature of transcendental reality
3. Samkhya/evolution of existence, nature of being, mental discrimination for perception of reality, rather than knowing through meditative experience
4. Yoga/practical techniques of meditation and self-control to attain the perception of self and reality, experiential learning
5. Vaisheshika/liberation by understanding all of existence in terms of the six primary categories
6. Myaya/rules, logic and rhetoric

Patanjali's eight limbs of yoga:

1. Samadhi/awakening and absorption in spirit
2. Dhyana/deep meditation
3. Dharana/one-pointed concentration
4. Pratyahar/synchronization of senses and thought
5. Pranayam/control of Prana (life force)
6. Asana/postures for health and meditation
7. Niyama/five disciplines (purity, contentment, purification, study, devotion)
8. Yama/five restraints (non-hurting, truthfulness, non-stealing, sensory control, non-possessiveness)

Disciplining the Mind and Aspects of the Elements

The negative mind is mastered with the five disciplines of Niyama and Yama.
The positive mind is mastered with Asanas and Pranayam.
The neutral mind is mastered with Pratyahar, Dharana, Dhyana, and Samadhi.

The five elements are balanced in the following ways:

1. Earth/habits - confronted by Yamas
2. Water/emotional impulse - guided by Niyamas
3. Fire/energy and the urge to do - tended by Asana
4. Air/sensitivity and feelings - directed by Pranayam
5. Ether/the creative inner-space - navigated with Pratyahar, Dharana, Dhyana, and Samadhi

I subscribe specifically to Kundalini (awareness energy) Yoga Meditation which is considered a Raj (king yoga) and incorporates all the aspects of yoga as a complete technology for the realization of wholeness and expanded consciousness. It is an amazing technology designed to cleanse, heal, and balance the entire human biofield, which includes the physical body, mind, emotions, soul, will, heart, glands, organs, and all systems....everything we know about and don't know about. It incorporates prescriptive yogic principles on all levels of our being directing the life force to achieve balance and excellence. Kundalini Yoga and meditation practice will be addressed further in the comprehensive healing systems section of the book.

Our complete existence is designed to constantly seek dynamic balance, homeostasis, when we are in motion, still or asleep. Daily physical exercise/movement of some sort is mandatory for our optimum health and well-being and it is far more than just physical fitness. This is also why any spiritual practice will include movement of some kind: physical, mental, emotional, spiritual and environmental.

The chart on the next page shows the pattern of movement along our energy arc lines and how it is stimulated by movement.

How Movement Causes Energy Flow - Esoteric Anatomy

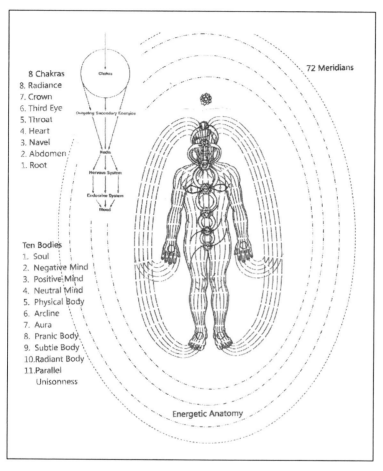

8 Chakras
8. Radiance
7. Crown
6. Third Eye
5. Throat
4. Heart
3. Navel
2. Abdomen
1. Root

Ten Bodies
1. Soul
2. Negative Mind
3. Positive Mind
4. Neutral Mind
5. Physical Body
6. Arcline
7. Aura
8. Pranic Body
9. Subtle Body
10. Radiant Body
11. Parallel
    Unisonness

72 Meridians

Energetic Anatomy

Chart from: *Esoteric Anatomy,* by Bruce Burger. Adapted by Merging Rivers Healing Practices 2008

Movement Resource Guide:

The Nia Technique, by Debbie Rosas and Carlos Rosas
Kundalini Yoga, by Skakti Parwha Kaur Kaulsa
Body Eloquence, by Nancy Mellon
Esoteric Anatomy, by Bruce Burger

7 - COMMUNICATION AND RELATIONSHIP - Our Reasons to Live

It is not what you say or do...it is your state of being that is your communication. Your very existence is your communication. Your relationship to anything including yourself is determined by the quality of your state of being . You are the underlying power and the energy dynamic. Thus, if it is change or control you seek, it must be of yourself.

-Andrea Becky 2010

There are volumes of written material on communication and relationship. Counselors, social workers, communication specialists, psychiatrists, psychologists, research scientists, life coaches, clergy, philosophers, programs and trainings specialize and focus on bettering communication and relationships offering methods and skills.

We will be looking at communication and relationship with an energetic approach which is significantly different from most traditional approaches. The focus will be on communication and relationship with the Self first and the energy dynamics and influences on communication and relationships with other people, places and things, spiritual aspects and proven communication basics and models.

The major influences in my life and in this energetic approach to communication and relationship have come from the unprecedented work of psychotherapist Carl Jung, John Bradshaw about addiction recovery, Marshall D. Rosenberg, Ph.D. about non-violent communication, Mira D. Kirshenbaum about couples therapy, Yogi Bhajan, Ph.D. about Kundalini teaching, and Barbara Ann Brennen about energy healing. You will find aspects of their work integrated and adapted in this chapter, and you will also find reading resources at the end of the chapter.

Anatomy of Communication and Relationship –
It Begins and Ends With You

Your relationships are your communication. How you relate to yourself, others and things is your communication. Your being is your communication. Communication is relationship in motion. Yes, there are skills and models that are helpful, but the state of your being will always talk louder than what you are saying or doing. If you are not aware of what establishes you in the present moment, you will be unable to communicate and relate in the ways you truly desire. You must at all times be aware of "where you are coming from." Know your intention, your emotional state of being and be established in your authentic self. Anything less than that will cause faulty communication and relationship issues. If you communicate something less than your truth, with pure intent, you cannot expect anything more in return.

Aspects of the energetic anatomy of communication and relationship are described by all of the universal laws. Energetic anatomy shows how pranic/unseen energy flows. Physical anatomy shows physical systems that are involved in the flow of blood, lymph, digestion, hormones, etc. and described by physical laws. To understand how they interrelate and are inseparable requires holistic knowledge, awareness and a strong felt sense.

When I ask people where communication and relationship happen, generally they reply that communication happens in your mind and relationship happens in your mind and heart. Energetically speaking, it happens in the space between where you are able to energetically connect indicated by the small circle in the drawing. The larger circle is the environment that influences the interaction. Please study the chart to get an idea of the influences in the dynamic and ever changing energetic structure of communication and relationship.

The Space Between Us

The space between us is sacred
And is of no time or space

It is not an obstacle but a fertile ground
With the promise of transformation, connection and freedom
A place of memory and reunion

It is not empty but full and rich with vibrating dynamic potential
There is the bright flame of healing warning that it could flicker
Without the fuel of honesty

Nothing can destroy it
And it allows us to flourish

But we must guard and preserve and nurture it
By allowing only love there.

-Andrea Becky 2001

One Chart Says It All - Relationship Happens in the Sacred Space Between

The key to the energetic approach to relationship is to be conscious and responsible about what you offer the relationship. If you do not put your authentic, honest, best self into the relationship, you will not like what is reflected back to you. The dynamic of meaningful and fulfilling relationship and communication is a circular, continuous and conscious and authentic exchange of personal truth. Anything less than that is a lie and the relationship cannot ultimately thrive or even survive. This level of authenticity and honesty is required no matter what other influences affect your communication and how you relate. This is an example of Self first responsibility. If an issue doesn't begin with authenticity and honesty, it often is not recoverable. Too much of that eventually erodes the communication and relationship.

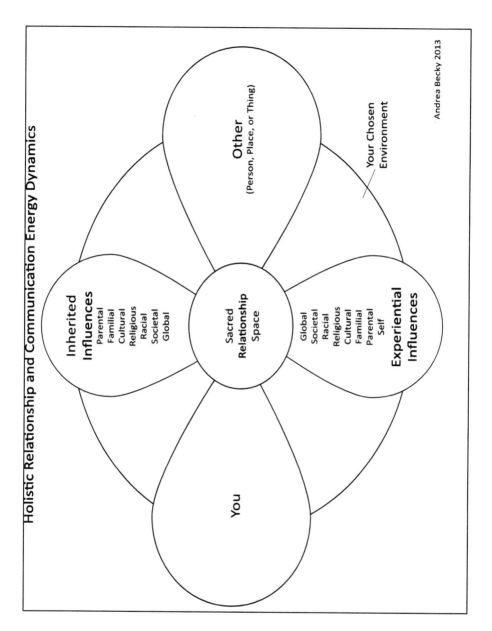

Holistic Relationship and Communication Energy Dynamics

Andrea Becky 2013

Other
(Person, Place, or Thing)

Your Chosen Environment

Inherited Influences
Parental
Familial
Cultural
Religious
Racial
Societal
Global

Sacred Relationship Space

Global
Societal
Racial
Religious
Cultural
Familial
Parental
Self
Experiential Influences

You

Full Spectrum Communication for Relationships of Your Dreams

Express what stirs within you and let your spirit speak.

-Andrea Becky

We are used to using our five senses, communicating with our minds and voices and words. Most of us know about body language, but that is usually somewhat unconscious. When communication and expression don't go well, we can feel unheard, judged or intimidated.

We know now that we are energy and information beings taking in and sharing energy and information in many dimensions. We do that using our senses, our ten bodies, eight chakras, 72,000 meridians. If we are not conscious of involving all of us, we may feel we are falling short of getting our message across and/or receiving other messages well.

Please review the chart below as a visual of what I call full spectrum communication. If you are open and willing to be honest and fully present when communicating, it becomes a more fulfilling experience. This is another reason to know who you are, what you believe in and what your deepest driving desires are.

In energetic communication, information is being projected through the chakras. Ideally, energy is flowing freely with no fear or hidden intentions, blocks or interruptions from all chakras to all chakras. Authenticity, trust, and vulnerability are terms that come to mind for most with this definition.

This is what full spectrum communication would look like:

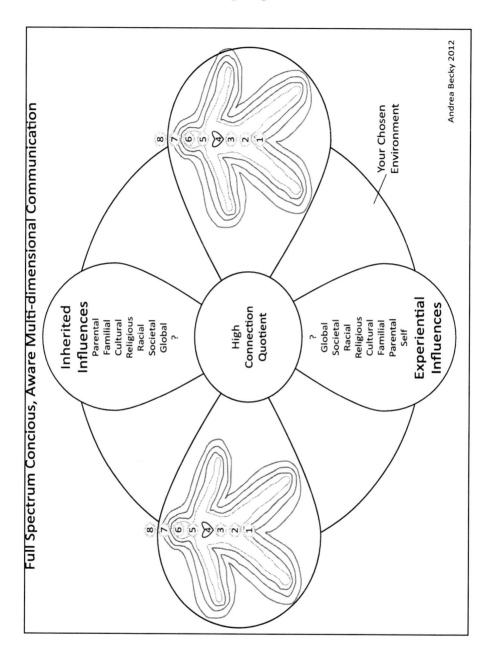

Full Spectrum Concious, Aware Multi-dimensional Communication

Inherited
Influences
Parental
Familial
Cultural
Religious
Racial
Societal
Global
?

High
Connection
Quotient

?
Global
Societal
Racial
Religious
Cultural
Familial
Parental
Self

Experiential
Influences

Your Chosen
Environment

Andrea Becky 2012

143

The Intense Power of Words

Words are fields of energy. The words you use are powerful and carry meaning far beyond their definition. So your state of being, what you say, how you say it and the words you use, deserve some serious thought if you want to improve your communication. Feel what you are saying or doing and choose your words for they are powerful beyond your imagination.

Words we use in place of feelings when...

Feeling powerless or victimized (another person is necessary to "feel" this way)

Abandoned
Abused
Attacked
Betrayed
Boxed-in
Bullied
Cheated
Coerced
Co-opted
Cornered
Distrusted
Interrupted
Intimidated
Let down
Manipulated
Misunderstood

Neglected
Overworked
Patronized
Pressured
Provoked
Put down
Rejected
Taken for granted
Threatened
Unappreciated
Unheard
Unseen
Unsupported
Unwanted
Used

NowOpp@ResolveConflict

For resolution, the question to ask is:

In what way am I _____ (the word you chose) - ing myself?

And how is the other person doing that to him/herself? This can lead to the real problem.

When you have the answer, start an activity that counters that.

Power words when our needs are being met:

Awesome	Nice
Bright	Optimistic
Carefree	Peaceful
Delightful	Quiet
Enthusiastic	Radiant
Fabulous	Secure
Glowing	Thankful
Hopeful	Upbeat
Invigorated	Vivacious
Joyful	Warm
Keyed-up	Yummy
Loving	Zestful
Mellow	

Power words when our needs are not being met:

Afraid	Lonely
Anxious	Lost
Bitter	Miserable
Blah	Meaningless
Chagrined	Nervous
Confused	Nauseated
Detached	Overwhelmed
Discouraged	Panicky
Embarrassed	Pessimistic
Empty	Resentful
Frightened	Restless
Frustrated	Skeptical
Gloomy	Sorry
Guilty	Terrified
Helpless	Tired
Hurt	Uneasy
Irritable	Unhappy
Invisible	Vexed
Jealous	Withdrawn
Jittery	

NowOpp@UniversalEnergyCorrection

The question...action here is: While rubbing you heart chakra saying, "Even though I feel _____, I completely love and accept myself." X3

When Communicating

Powerless Words

I am trying
I guess
When
If or when
But
Always
Never
Because

Should, shouldn't
Don't
Have to
Can't
Maybe
If, when, kind of, sort of
Whatever, I don't know and
    don't care

Powerful Words

I am or I am not...
I feel or know or have a
    sense that
Now
Now And Often
Rarely
No apologies, no explanations
Could

Choose not to
Get to
Can find out
It is possible now
I have a sense that

Outdated Defense Systems - Living In the Past

We learn at young ages that we need defense systems and mechanisms to avoid hurt and embarrassment. The problem is that we mature and our lives change and most often the defense systems don't work anymore, and frustration, misunderstanding and possible hopelessness sets in.

Defense systems create energetic states that are not at all conducive to full spectrum communication.

The leading edge energy healer and teacher, Barbara Ann Brennen, in her book, *Light Emerging*, shows the image of what various defense positions look like. Just by browsing the chart below, you can sense communication and relationship is deterred by these states.

Energetic Defense Systems

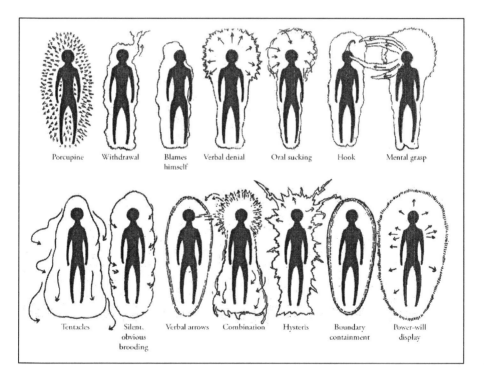

From *Light Emerging*, by Barbara Ann Brennan

147

Skewed Defense Systems – Living In Fear

This work on full spectrum communication and relationship began out of fear and frustration and a sense of hopelessness with someone I was attempting to help. It was someone who was in traditional psychiatric therapy but was still deeply struggling with grief and drug and alcohol addiction and who I will call "Pat."

This was a fairly long-term circumstance that was steadily deteriorating. I was concerned for this person's safety at this point in terms of a possible over-dose or driving accident. When I attempted to intervene and or counsel Pat, who would slip into drug-induced psychosis, she would double-over, hold her midsection with her arms, moan and say "Stop, you are hurting me!" This happened two or three times and I was baffled. Of course, the "communication" would end there and the hopelessness would set in.

By a total "coincidence," while in a metaphysical book store in Los Angeles, the person walking down the aisle of health and healing books knocked a book off the shelf unknowingly with his backpack. He turned to pick it up and I told him I would get it. It was Barbara Brennen's book, *Light Emerging*. It had fallen in an open position and as I glanced at it, I realized it was about a person's energy field when in a state of psychosis. I was stunned, but this kind of thing had happened before and I knew it was a gift.

The energy field was asymmetrical and blown out up to the right much like the withdrawal field in the chart above...and, there was a big hole in the field over the abdominal area! Also, in the description was that communicating with a person in this state normally would cause distress, and to direct your communication energetically above the persons head some distance. I stood there in the aisle in somewhat of a trance – time had stood still – trying to grasp the miracle of the synchronicity, but energized with new hope.

Next time I saw Pat, I applied the gift of new knowledge and awareness I had received. It was difficult not to fall into my old patterns of making eye contact and speaking heart to heart and I felt uncomfortable, however...it worked! Pat looked up and made eye contact with me for the first time in a long time. She didn't double over and she didn't reply or communicate with words, but she showed interest and response. That was enough and that moment was the beginning of her ultimate recovery.

What are your automatic conditioned or habitual or skewed defensive responses? Identify what applies to you and/or circle words that describe you in most stressful situations. Be as honest as you can with yourself. When under stress or pressed or feeling attacked, I tend to:

_____ 1. Get mentally confused, irrational or distracted

_____ 2. Take blame, abuse, fault and/or to try to make it right

_____ 3. Become the victim of injustice, unfairness or bullying

_____ 4. Get irritated, angry or hostile and intimidate or take control

_____ 5. Feel competitive and fight overtly or covertly

_____ 6. Become righteous and blaming, disgusted

_____ 7. Become manipulative and slippery, sabotage or undermine

_____ 8. Withdraw, disavow or wish it would go away

_____ 9. Close down and act like nothing is happening

_____ 10. Other _____

_____ 11. Accept, assess and allow a solution to evolve from knowing within there is a way through every problem. (If you checked #10, Congratulations! If not, this is the goal and read on.)

Having identified your learned defensive behavior is the first step in realizing it keeps you from meaningful and fulfilling full spectrum communication and relationship. Defense mechanisms are held in place by fear and resentment. The second step is to replace that defensive process with responsible, safe and effective communication and consequently a better relationship with yourself and others and things. A good place to start is to own your needs and desires and speaking for yourself without blame or pity. A very well-known and practiced method to do this is to use "I statements." Below are rules for response-able communication. Look them over and begin practicing them. When you take responsibility and feel what you communicate, it creates sanity and value and power within to what you are saying, and to others. These are truly golden rules.

Being Self-Response-Able

1. Use I statements and speak personally and specifically rather than generally and abstractly.
2. Listen to your inner voice and prompting. Become aware of when you are prompted to speak, move, or express, and when you are not.
3. When you feel moved, speak thoughtfully and with care—avoid abstract conceptual language and stories.
4. Understand the value of silence in communication. Become comfortable with silence...your own and others.
5. Be present emotionally, whether you are speaking or not. Feel what you are feeling.
6. Listen carefully and with respect to what another person is saying. Respect their process.
7. Don't try to fix someone else or give advice, this process is about you and what you are feeling as you sit in silence and listen to internal and external cues.
8. Be aware of your own barriers, such as prejudices, expectations, ideologies, judgments or need to control, which are obstacles to connectedness.
9. Stay in touch as deeply as possible with your feelings without self-judgment and without blaming others.
10. State your name prior to speaking – this allows you to own what you say.
11. Speak from your heart, not your head or thoughts or beliefs.
12. Listen from your heart.
13. Trust the Process.
14. Respect confidentiality. What is spoken and experienced in the group should remain with the group and not discussed outside the group.
15. Be inclusive.

Conscious Communication and Relationship

- Know what energetic state is establishing you in the present moment.
- Be aware of what energetic state is establishing others in the present moment.
- Always be aware of where you are coming from, what your intention is, and where your intentions are taking you.
- Hear and choose your words knowing they are powerful beyond your imagination.
- Know who you are and be your authentic self at all costs. Give the gift of truth.
- Make your goal to release all defense mechanisms that get in the way of satisfying full spectrum communication and relationships.

A Basic and Sound Communication Model to Practice

Tone Choice Established in?	Communication	Action
Compassion Joy	What is really bothering me?	CIA *Introspection*
Control Neediness	When I (see, hear, feel) you _____ ...	*Your perception*
Anger Fear Sarcasm	I feel (mad, sad, glad, scared...)	*Identify and expressing your emotions/ feelings*
Grief Hate	What I imagine is _____ ...	*Stating your interpretation*
Sadness Envy	What I would like from you is _____ .	*Expressing your needs*
Greed Regret	What are your needs about this _____ ?	*Inviting useful dialogue*
Guilt	Can we agree to _____ ?	*Making a cooperative creative contract*
	Thank you for hearing me.	*Vibrating Gratitude*

Use any part or the whole sequence as is or modified for the situation. Speak your truth. Speak from the heart. Be open to any positive outcome. All tones are ultimately aimed at yourself even though you may be directing or projecting them on another person, thing, or idea.

Love Thyself... - The Bible
To Thine Own Self Be True - Shakespeare

Kundalini Yoga Rules of Communication

- You are communicating for a better tomorrow, not to spoil today
- Whatever you are going to say is going to live forever, and we all have to live through it
- One wrong word said can do much more wrong than you can even imagine or even estimate
- Words spoken are a chance for communication. Don't turn them into a war
- When you communicate, you have to communicate again. Don't make the road rough

Relationship and Communication Resource Guide:

The Aquarian Teacher, by Yogi Bhajan, Ph.D.
Seven Spiritual Laws of Success, by Deepak Chopra
Healing the Shame That Binds You, by John Bradshaw
The Work, by Byron Katie
Light Emerging, by Barbara Brennen
Too Good to Leave, Too Bad to Stay, by Mira Kirshenbaum
Nonviolent Communication: A Language of Life, by Marshall D. Rosenberg, Ph.D.
The Psychology of Kundalini Yoga, by Carl G. Jung

Section Five

Timely Evolved Perspectives for Healing

The Best Kept Secret of Healing Now – Energy Psychology

Unusual, Unbelievable and It Works

Energy Psychology is the perfect union of the best of psychology, Kinesiology and the best ancient healing technology to create a body knowledge, techniques and therapies that very effectively and quickly clear, balance and restore human functioning. This approach to healing often works when nothing else has. This evidence-based world of healing provides profound relief and sustainable transformative healing in this world of relentless stress and challenges. The results of treatment are so impressive in most cases, it sometimes causes a belief gap from the point of view of traditional medicine and even from the client who has come to expect reoccurring issues. However, the outcomes are undeniable as reported by those who use these methods around the world as clients and as practitioners and professionals expanding their practices, and world service organizations deepening their ability to help.

Clinical and research-based outcomes have shown Energy Psychology Methods help alleviate many issues associated with Post Traumatic Stress Disorder, anxiety, phobias, depression, addictions, weight management, pain, emotional turmoil, and have been shown to support improvement in school, sports and work performance.

Energy Psychology is an integrative holistic approach in that treatment methods and techniques seek relief from the source or interruption in the energy system contributing to the issues, and includes consideration of the multi-layered interconnection of all systems of the body and field, as well as the proper flow of energy through the energy system.

This is an empowering, comprehensive, complex family of healing modalities with many deep roots from proven healing methods. And, that being said, some modalities are so simple they can be taught to children for independent use. Examples of the many methods included in the Energy Psychology family are Emotional Freedom Technique (EFT), Thought Field Therapy (TFT), Tapas Acupressure Technique (TAT), Comprehensive Energy Psychology (CEP), Matrix Energetics, Soul Detective Work, Energy Medicine, Emotional Fitness

System, Be Set Free Fast (BSFF), Neuro Emotional Technique (NET), Healing From the Body Level Up (HBLU), Seemorg Matrix Work, Energetic Diagnostic and Treatment Methods (EDXTM), and numerous other methods.

Meridian-based therapies with their ancient wisdom and leading edge scientific roots come from a huge body of knowledge. Please look over some basic premises of the work, learn one of the leading methods and deepen your understanding even more of this amazing, relatively new body of extraordinary healing possibilities.

Basic Premises of Energy Psychology

- Energy Psychology incorporates and integrates leading edge tools for healing and transformation based on the most ancient healing practices and contemporary scientific discoveries.
- Basic discovery statement is that stress or discomfort or disease is caused by an interruption in the energy system that can be identified and resolved for the proper flow of energy.
- The main roots of Energy Psychology are Applied Kinesiology, Behavioral Kinesiology, Psychology, Neurophysiology, Ayurveda, Yoga, Meditation, Nursing, Neuro Linguistic Programming, Physical Therapy, Chiropractic, Oriental Medicine, Hypnosis, Transpersonal Work, Shamanism, Scientific Research and Quantum Physics.
- It is a non-exclusive approach that can be applied to anything.
- We are energy beings (electromagnetic energy and light) and have an energy blueprint and infrastructure, which interplays with our cells, glands, organs, emotions, thoughts, beliefs and actions.
- By influencing the flow of energy through our energy centers (Chakras) pathways (Meridians) and layers of bodies (Biofield), we can affect cleansing, balancing, enhancing our health on all levels and our sense of well-being.
- This origin-seeking, homeopathic, solution-oriented, vibrational or energetic approach works quickly and usually results in sustainable personal change, allows personal growth and self realization.

How Do Energy Psychology Modalities Work?

Holistic approaches to healing recognize the interconnected and multi-layered, multidimensional nature of the human as a whole. The sciences of psychoneuroimmunology, epi-genetics, interpersonal neurobiology and neuroplasticity support the premise of the holistic energetic approach.

It appears that the interrelated effect of focusing attention on specific memories, beliefs, emotions and/or experiences while learning and practicing skills to influence the flow of energy in the energy system to resolve disruptions and normalize the system functions, result in changes that typically transcend the normal ability to change with conscious effort. In fact, it is common for spontaneous resolution of negative thoughts, emotions, and memories that many times have been long-term problems or conflicts. This has created quite a belief gap in the traditional fields of psychology and medicine.

Because the results affect the flow of the life-force throughout the entire field, it appears that all aspects of the field, physical and non-physical are included in the resolution. Clients often report improvement in their self image, health, relations with others and interaction with work and social environments.

Emotional Freedom at Your Fingertips!

We will use Emotional Freedom Technique (EFT), which I consider a "gold standard" for Energy Psychology. The technique can be initially self-taught and used immediately to experience the results. And, it can be used as a therapeutic tool by healing professionals. It is a simple and comprehensive tapping technique developed by founder, Gary Craig in the 1990's. Also, much of the research done in this field has used EFT, and it is especially suitable for a Now Opp.

A Note About Side Effects of Using Energy Psychology Techniques:

- The worst thing that can happen is nothing.
- Because EP Methods influence the flow of energy, you may experience feelings of tingling, release, lightness and even some slight disorientation from the correction in energy flow in your field. This is temporary.
- You may experience a sense of relief and/or of joy for "no apparent reason."
- You may feel somewhat lost without the nagging problem, thought, emotion or belief demanding your attention or plaguing you any longer.
- Your perception of other people, your environment and/or yourself may be more pleasant and interesting, and/or feel safer.
- It may seem comical that you cannot access the negativity released any longer.
- Meridian-based treatment has been shown to help with a long list of issues: abundance, weight loss, business and career goals, emotional challenges, children's behavior, relationship issues, anger management, stress management, depression, anxiety, insomnia, severe trauma, addictions, sexual abuse, phobias, physical distress, allergies, migraines, pain management, chronic fatigue, hypertension, fibromyalgia, cancer, muscular dystrophy, Parkinson's, cystic fibrosis.

NowOpp@EFT

This instructional session is an opportunity to get a firsthand experience with EFT. This is a practice that can change your life… turn the tide of negativity and emotional turmoil. This is a tool you will want to know and have to apply to situations in your life.

The Emotional Freedom Technique Practice

It is not necessary to use the whole technique all the time. Choosing to use it and pure intention to heal are the empowering factors. It is more effective if done according to directions; however, any attempt will be useful and will not cause any harm. Simply do your best and try it on everything!

To Start: Take a deep breath and be sure you are adequately hydrated.

Bring a problem, thought, emotion or experience to mind that is bothering you. Think about it in detail and subjectively rate its intensity on a scale of one to ten (one is annoying and ten is extremely distressing). Refer to the chart on the next page for clarity.

Step one: Set up points - You may experiment with and choose from three locations.

(This is an adaptation from my treatment experience; Classic EFT usually uses the Karate Point or Sore Spots)

1. Karate Point- The outside (little finger side) edge of either hand and tapping with three or four finger pads of the opposite hand while saying the affirmation below.
2. Sore Spots - Location different on each person - Press with pads of index and middle fingers in a small circular motion while saying the affirmation below.
3. Heart Center - With an open palm of either hand, rub the heart center in a clockwise direction (up to the left and down and around to the right) while saying the affirmation below.

Affirmation: "Even though I have this (problem, feeling, condition), I completely accept and love myself." (c.a.l.m.) Repeat the affirmation three times.

Step two: Tapping Sequence - Tap five to seven times on each acupoint with the pads of the index and middle fingers on points 1 through 11 while repeating words that describe your feelings about the issue or simply thinking about the issue you have chosen. Use both hands on points 1-7 and the opposite hand on points 8-11.

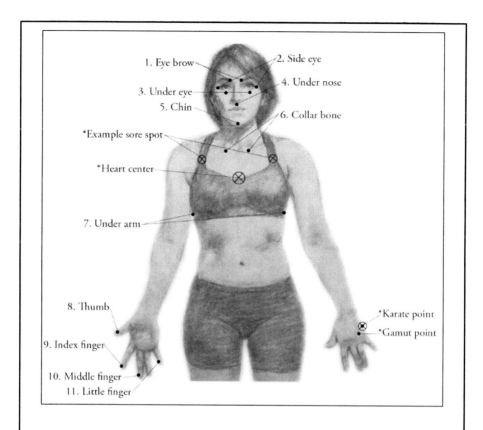

1. Eye brow
2. Side eye
3. Under eye
4. Under nose
5. Chin
6. Collar bone
*Example sore spot
*Heart center
7. Under arm
8. Thumb
9. Index finger
10. Middle finger
11. Little finger
*Karate point
*Gamut point

Step three: 9 Gamut Process

Tap with two or three finger pads on the back of the opposite hand between ring and little finger knuckles continuously and complete the following actions:

1. Close eyes
2. Open eyes
3. Look down to the right with eyes
4. Look down left with eyes
5. Roll eyes in a circle right
6. Roll eyes in a circle left
7. Hum a tune
8. Count to 5 quickly
9. Hum a tune

Step four: Repeat the sequence of step two and complete with a deep breath.

Step five: Rate the problem again on the scale of 1-10
   Is your subjective rating lower? If not, take some deep breaths and be sure you are hydrated and try it again. If it is lower, see step six.

Step six: Subsequent rounds
   In subsequent rounds, the setup affirmation and reminder phrase are adjusted to reflect the fact that you are addressing the *remaining* problem, feeling, or condition. Continue until it is resolved to a one or zero rating.

Step seven: Be aware of changes in how you related to the issue you worked on. With Energy Psychology, one of the measures is how the healing plays out in your life. Over time, be aware of how circumstances are different involving the issue you worked on. Congratulations and enjoy.

Step eight: Tapping in the Positive Affirmations using Positive EFT. Now you may wish to install positive affirmations regarding your issue, using positive affirmations that reflect your desired circumstances. For example, I am a joyful confident person. I enjoy good health. I feel tranquil and loved.

Using EFT – Three Case Examples

I Do Something Else When Everyone Goes Hiking

Sally is an intelligent and athletic fifty-four year old woman. When her friends asked her to go hiking in the mountains, she always had an excuse. No one knew that Sally was deathly afraid of heights. She came to an Emotional Fitness retreat and the first evening, I asked for a volunteer with a phobia to demonstrate EFT. Sally volunteered. She shared her lifetime fear, and how silly it was she was afraid of hiking in hills and mountains, and was at a destination where that is one of the main activities.

As we discussed her fear, she began to have the actual physical responses of anxiety and fear just talking about it. I asked her to rate the impact of the fear on a scale of 1-10 and she said it was an eight, and muscle testing confirmed that. We proceeded with the EFT protocol and saying words like this fear, this anxiety, this resentment, this sadness, this embarrassment, this shame, and this limitation and so on as we tapped.

We did one full round of EFT and Sally expressed a feeling of relief and that it was harder to access the fear. I asked her to rate the fear now, and she said it was three with surprise in her voice. We did a subsequent round using the phrase, this remaining fear, etc. At that point, Sally was euphoric and said, "I don't think I am afraid anymore," in disbelief. She rated the impact now at a one, but the muscle testing validation indicated it was zero.

The next morning we had a retreat hike planned. Sally joined us and was like a little girl on a new adventure and hiked comfortably. The whole group was elevated.

I Can't Camp with My family

Mar Dee was working the weekend because the rest of her family had gone camping. I asked her if she didn't like camping. She said, "Oh no, I love camping, but I am too afraid of the critters." I asked her what she meant by critters and she said she was terribly afraid of mice, rats, ground squirrels and anything like that. She shared, "I can't even look at a picture of them. If I go camping, I get hysterical if I see a critter and everybody gets upset and sometimes I end up going home."

I offered her a consultation to work on the critter phobia and she agreed she would like that. We completed two rounds of EFT and she indicated she felt differently about the critters. From a distance, I showed her a book I had with pictures of mice. She said, I think I can hold that, and she did! She was amazed and in disbelief because this had been problem for her as long as she could remember. We agreed that I would see her the next day and see how she was doing.

I borrowed a pet mouse from the little boy next door and took it with me in a small cage to see Sally.

She said she really felt different. I told her I had a live mouse in a cage in my car and asked her if she would like to see it. She hesitated and then said, "I think so..." We went out to the car. She stood her distance while I got the cage out of the car. She walked towards it step by step and kept saying... "No way! No-way!" I'm really not afraid of it. She even petted his head.

In two weeks, Sally called me to report she had gone along on the neighborhood family camping trip and had a wonderful time. She said her family and the neighbors couldn't believe it and thought it was a miracle...and it does seem miraculous indeed.

Green and Sick with Betrayal and Jealously

A friend of Andean had recommended she see me. Andean was nearly destroyed by the discovery of her husband's long-term affair with her best friend. She had lost weight and was on medication for high anxiety.

We scheduled an appointment and when she came, she was actually shaking with anxiety, fear, jealously, resentment and sense of betrayal. She briefly related the circumstances and began crying while at the same time feeling anger and resentment and jealously that she said was "taking her down." We took some time to calm down a bit with deep breaths and drinking some water, and then began the EFT therapy. We did one round which was intense as she said the words that described her feelings as we tapped. We paused at the end of the round, did some more deep breathing and drank some more water.

Andean sat calmly in the chair, exhausted and "feeling blank." After a few moments, she said, "That really helped! This is the first time I have not felt totally consumed by all that has happened." We continued with another round using the remaining phrase and again paused and rested. Her face and posture had changed and she said she felt so much lighter and was actually trying to access the jealously and anxiety and couldn't.

She said it felt "far away." This is a common comment after a session. We talked a bit and discussed what she was going to do from here and agreed to follow-up in a few weeks.

In two weeks, Andean emailed me with the message that she had a new lease on life and, although she was still shocked, she feels calm and confident. She is planning a divorce, which she had actually wanted for a couple of years, and was going back to school to finish her masters in art therapy. She said she was happier than she had been for several years.

The Complex, Interrelated Nature of Energy Treatment Points

For your interest and to raise your awareness about interconnectedness of the unseen energy body and the physical body, the drawing below shows tapping acupoint locations, correlating main meridian, organs, chakras and emotions. (For a more left brain version please see the chart on the next page.)

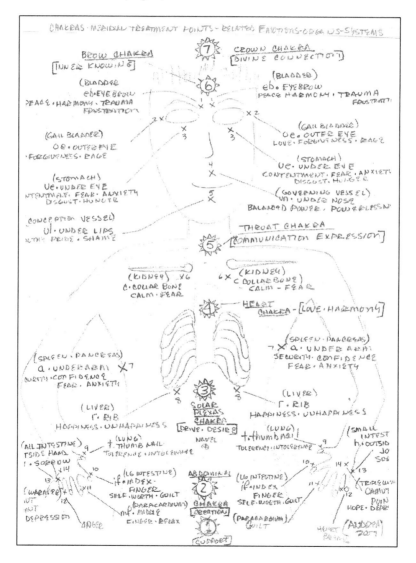

Acupoint Treatment Area Location	ID	Meridian	Negative Emotions and States of Being	Positive Emotions and States of Being
Eyebrow	eb	Bladder	Trauma, frustration, impatience, restlessness	Peace, harmony, calm
Outer Eye	oe	Gallbladder	Rage, fury, wrath	Love, forgiveness
Under Eye	e	Stomach	Fear, anxiety, bitterness, greed, depravation	Contented and tranquil
Under Nose	un	Governor Vessel	Powerlessness, inferiority, embarrassment	Confidence and in creative power
Under Lips	ul	Conception Vessel	Shame, undeserving	Secure, healthy self image, unique
Collarbone	c	Kidney	Fear, anxiety, indecision	Self assured
Under Arm	Ua	Spleen	Fear, worry about future	Secure, faith in future
Rib	R	Liver	Unhappy and angry	Happy, cheerful, joyous
Thumb	T	Lung	Judgment, contempt, prejudice, scorn, disdain	Neutral, forgiving, compassionate
Index Finger	If	Large Intestine	Guilt	Self knowledge, loved
Middle Finger	Mf	Pericardium	Jealousy, regret, remorse, stubbornness, tension	Ability to relax, release, understand, balanced
Little Finger	Lf	Heart	Anger	Acceptance
Karate/Side of Hand	sh (k)	Small Intestine	Sadness and sorrow	Joy, understanding
Gamut/Back of Hand	bh (g)	Triple Energizer	Depression, despair, grief, hopelessness, loneliness	Light, knowing, satisfied
Chakra Location	**ID**	**Regulation Aspect**	**Negative States of Being**	**Positive States of Being**
Above Head	Divine 8	Divinity	Depression, lonliness	Bliss
Crown/Top of Head	Crown 7	Divine Connection	Depression, despair	Connected
Center Forehead	Intuitive 6	Intuition	Rigid	Flexible
Neck/Throat	Throat 5	Communication	Suppressed	Free, spontaneous
Center of Chest	Heart 4	Love, harmony	Defensive	Open, calm, loving
Just Above Navel	Solar Plexas 3	Desire, expression	Thwarted, useless	Productive, motivated
Just Below Navel	Abdominal 2	Procreativity	Bored, uncreative, alone	Interactive, creative
Over Pubic Bone	Sacral 1	Support, nurturing	Unsupported, depraved	Supported, strong

Interrelatedness of Acupoints, Meridians, Chakras, Emotions, States of being and the Physical Systems

Summary and Resources

This is only a brief introduction to a profound and bountiful body of knowledge and opportunity for extraordinary healing. You can learn more for your own healing and if you choose to learn and expand your ability to teach and help others. Please take note of the suggested resources listed below.

Energy Psychology Resource Guide:

EFT & Energy Psychology, Tap Into Your Body's Energy to Change Your Life for the Better, by David Feinstein, Donna Eden & Gary Craig

The Promise of Energy Psychology, by David Feinstein, Donna Eden, Gary Craig and Mike Bowen

The Energy of Belief, by Sheila Bender and Mary Sise

Energy Medicine: Balancing Your Body's Energies for Optimal Health, Joy and Vitality, by Donna Eden and David Feinstein

The EFT Manual, by Gary Craig

Energy Psychology, Innovations in Psychology, by Fred Gallo

Energy Psychology Interactice Self-help Guide, by David Feinstein and Candace Pert

Heal Yourself with Emotional Freedom Technique, by John Freedom

When Three Dimensions Are Not Enough – Multidimensional Healing

Having lived on the edge of multi-dimensional reality as long as I could remember, and being familiar with receiving energy and information from other than the five senses, it's no surprise I was destined to travel deep into the "unknown" and experience the "un-thought-of."

I will say up front that this area of my life has been a particularly amazing adventure and extremely validating. Adventurous, because I can clearly remember when I was "afraid" of the unknown, death and the spirit world, and when only science fiction allowed the wandering of my mind into the "unimaginable." Validating, because all that I imagined about the spirit world has been shown to me to be true.

It also has given me a context to compare how really out of balance aspects of life on Earth really are. It is heartening, as well, to be able to be in the pure and judgeless energy and information fields I have had the blessing of experiencing. I no longer need to take anyone else's word for the nature of "the other side." And, by the way, it really isn't "the other side"... it is just another dimension. It is where answers lie that we cannot fathom and yet make perfect sense.

We can change the past and the future there, heal trauma there, and say what we didn't say or couldn't say and find answers to old unanswered questions. We can communicate with loved ones who have passed, and in fact, I frequently still get very specific loving guidance from my Mother who passed in 2002. That "world" is consistent, congruent, fluid and communicative 24/7/366.

Something else I didn't expect is all of history exists in the other dimensions (jury is out on all futures, except in terms of all potentiality and alternate futures), and other dimensions seem to include other planets, solar systems, and I am coming to believe, other galaxies. "All Is One Unending One" seems to be infinitely true. Experiences and shared information from other dimensions by "non-humans" also seem to confirm possible alternate beginnings when compared with supporting archeological findings and theories.

With our digital, energy everywhere, all things are possible world, the collective belief gap is definitely narrowing. Mine has all but disappeared, and that is a source of comfort. Working in other and parallel dimensions is extremely validating and the information and resolutions experienced are ambassadors for understanding and acceptance of our multidimensional nature.

A Word about Past Lives

My attitude about past lives is based on my belief that Souls are infinite, and so repeated incarnations seem perfectly normal to me. Even if you don't "believe in past lives," just the fact that energy and information is passed on in DNA and genes, can be a sort of past life influence. Also, the fact that I have dreamed past or parallel lives and have seen direct correlations of unsolved issues in past lives affecting this life, makes me a believer. In any case, we do know that "past life" healing can discover and resolve issues in this life that seem to have no origin in this life. I choose to just do the healing and enjoy the results and don't have to know if past lives are real or not. The results are real.

Slipping Into a Past Reality

I was so used to pursuing knowledge and experience in other dimensions, I was really taken aback when suddenly and unknowingly I found myself in a past life...twice in the same day in the same place. We had taken four days to complete the Machu Picchu Trail and complete the Incan Initiation with an Incan Shaman. It was an amazing, surreal adventure. On the last day, we were in Machu Picchu completing the initiation ceremonies as we went from feature to feature of the magnificent structures high in the Andes of Peru.

We were in front of the terraced gardens as our Shaman guide told us of the once elaborate plants, vegetables and herbs that were grown there. Suddenly, my whole reality shifted, my knees were weak and I began to shake and visualize me as about a five year-old girl playing and helping my mother in the second garden level up from where we were standing. I lost total awareness of my current body and environment and the entire landscape was from another time. Tears were streaming down my face and I was barely able to stand. My husband held me up and asked what was wrong. I could barely talk to say some feeble things like, "I was here a long time ago. It was so beautiful and I was so happy." As the current reality faded back in, I just felt shaken and sad. We sat down for a few minutes and had some water and then continued on with our initiation tour.

We continued to the temple area where there is a triangular rock carved altar sometimes identified as a sacrificial altar. As we approached, it happened again. My awareness of myself and the current surroundings shifted into another time. I was very frightened. I was a young boy and I had been chosen to be sacrificed. I couldn't show emotion for this was an honor. I could see my mother standing in the background and my father up ahead. The intensity and fear repelled me from the dimension and I popped back out.

I have since done energy work to release the fear and confused emotions from that life. However, as I write about this, I can still sense remnants of that life. I have not slipped into a past life since, but have intentionally gone there. I believe that happened to inform me of parallel and past life energy.

Another Perception and Life Changing Experience

It was November 1, 1984 and it was Dia de los Muertos, (Day of the Dead). We were in Oaxaca, Mexico. At that time, I was an art consultant and in Mexico on business. The business was of purchasing the beautiful Animales de Medera, (animals carved of wood). Our whole family would go on these buying trips and it had been a wonderful endeavor. We were able get to know the artists and their families. We played basketball in the park with them and took Polaroid pictures that we gave to them. Many of them had never seen a photo of themselves. Each time we returned they thanked us for the photos which were displayed prominently in their homes and on the church bulletin board. They were gracious and hospitable and this year, they had invited us to their celebration of Dia de los Muertos, the celebration of those who had passed in their families and village. This is their version of Halloween and All Saints Day, and not at all comparable to ours. It is a grand two-day celebration.

We had spent the afternoon experiencing the festivities, sipping the wonderful Champarrado (Mexican Hot Chocolate) and being offered Chapulines (deep fried grasshoppers), a grand delicacy collected and cooked especially for the holiday.

All the preparations had been completed and it was time to go to the cemetery where the celebration would continue over night. Each family took photos, toys, the favorite food and tequila and music and clothes of the deceased as gifts for their visit of the dead ones. We had blankets, chairs and small tables to put all the food on at the grave sites.

The cemetery was full with the families of the village, music, food, gifts...and the spirits of the deceased. With no warning or intention, suddenly I could see them! In the candle light and with all the villagers, I had to blink my eyes to tell the difference at times. They would fade into sight and out. When the shock wore off a bit, I was also surprised that I wasn't frightened. Fully immersed in the culture and the festival, it seemed perfectly normal. I asked some of our friends if they could see the spirits and they replied with gusto "Si, si, si! Usted también?" I just nodded my head like it wasn't any big thing and didn't say much more. Even though I wasn't frightened, I was still a bit stunned. The sweetness of the reunions and the melding of dimensions and remembering was deeply emotional. I was struck by their ability to bridge the gap of the living and the dead, grief and celebration and joy. Most of the families stayed until dawn and we went back to our hotel room.

I didn't say much to anyone for fear that they would think I was hallucinating and it still was a very sacred and surreal experience. I did, however, begin reading and studying various mediums because the experience was so impactful.

Years went by, and I didn't have another experience like that, but I did decide to start training in multi-cultural and multi-dimensional studies with my dear friend, shaman and spiritual adventurer, Betina. For four years, we took courses as we had time. The training was transforming and I felt like I was being gently molded for the next phase of my life. We learned to command light and energy in many ways for healing ourselves, others and the environment and even the galaxy. My beliefs and imagination were stretched to the max. And little did I know this was just the beginning.

A particularly noticeable turning point was learning some chakra past lives healing training that used hands over the field and intuiting through the energy of the palms information about a past life. We would determine the age, sex and time of the life, the trauma at death, heal it and clear the field. In the beginning, I can remember thinking I was just making it up, but with practice and the accompanying undeniable healing results, I began to trust the process and the way information could be felt and interpreted through my palms, be healed, released and help with issues in this life. An adjunct to that training was the understanding and ability to help a dying person's soul leave the body and transcend with chakra healing work. We just learned the technique "in case we needed it." Naively, I thought I never would.

Stepping Into Possibilities

I fell asleep on the takeoff of the plane going home from a ski trip in Colorado. Ski trips were fun, but never relaxing and I was tired. We had a layover in Las Vegas. My Mom was ninety-one and she had been failing in health and was more on my mind than usual. I called my sister from Las Vegas and she confirmed what I was feeling which was I should probably plan to go to Salt Lake City soon. That is where my Mom lived. Instead of taking the second leg of the flight home to San Diego, we booked a flight to Salt Lake arriving four hours later. The children flew from San Diego arriving the next day.

I was so thankful I had a chance to spend some time with my Mom. Even though she was quite sedated, we still communicated well. The priest had given her last rites and had returned to the parish. Hospice was there. It was reassuring, and one of the hospice staff played the harp, which was sobering and comforting. The harp player left, the rest of the family was in the kitchen and I found myself alone sitting by my Mother's bed with her. She looked very peaceful. She and I knew this was the end and the time of her passing.

Suddenly, I remembered the training for helping the spirit leave the body. It was so difficult for me to accept that her death was eminent and that I had the ability, authority or the audacity to think I should help her transcend. And then a voice said, "This is no accident, help her." I hesitantly stood up. I asked her if she wanted help, and I felt her say yes. I, still hesitantly, placed my hands palms down about eight inches above her chakras using a counter clockwise circular motion to the left from her first chakra to the eighth chakra and up and away above her head. I repeated this three times as instructed and said prayers for her safe and blessed passage. I stood by her bed for a long time still feeling trepidation about my role in my Mother's passing.

Two hours and fifteen minutes later, my Mother officially passed. The death of any loved one, and particularly a parent at any age, is a deep source of retrospection and realization of our own mortality. My sister, brother and I were now the "front line of the family." Making funeral plans, plans for her belongings and fulfilling her last wishes was bitter sweet, and her long and purposeful life passed deeply through my consciousness.

About six weeks later, a friend of mine recommended a psychic intuitive by the name of Tara to me. With all that had happened in the past year, I decided to go to her. Because I am basically a skeptic, when I made an appointment, I made sure she knew nothing about me or even who recommended me.

I arrived at her very warm and attractive home and walked up to the door and raised my hand to use the door knocker. The door flew open and a bubbly blond-haired woman exclaimed, "I am so glad you are here, your Mother has been here for hours!"

Tara invited me in and we sat in a very pleasant room for our consultation. She began by saying, "Let me just start with the message from your Mother. She wants to thank you for helping her leave." My heart filled and tears of joy and relief came to my eyes. Tara continued, "She also wants you to know she has been trying to get your attention with all the birds, wondered if you noticed them." I certainly had, many experiences of birds flying very near, one that was trying to stand on the round doorknob of our front door, two in the house, one of which was a humming bird that dropped a feather as it flew back out. I still have the feather. And at that moment, a bird was attempting to perch on the very small and slanted brick window sill outside the window we were sitting by. We both laughed and Tara proceeded to describe my Mom to the tee. We talked about many other aspects of my life. From that moment on, my doubt subsided and the door to the spirit world was open and I have gratefully, I have been able to maintain open communication with my Mother.

A Series of Related Incidents

A year passed and I continued to train in multicultural and multidimensional healing endeavors. I also began teaching the healing practices of meditation and Ayurveda at a wonderful destination resort called, Red Mountain, in Ivins, Utah and developed my business called, Merging Rivers Healing Practices, all with recommendations from my former teacher, my guides and my Mother's messages.

I realized that a pathway to opening the psyche and the heart and will was through the emotions and formulated my presentations around that idea. I became interested in meridian-based modalities and self trained with DVD's CD's and the *Manual for Emotional Freedom Technique*. I was astounded with the application to the long list of emotionally-based issues and learned muscle testing at a seminar with Brad Nelson, author of *Emotion Code*. That is what led up to the development of my curriculum integrating energy healing, kundalini yoga and meditation, intuitive reading, movement therapy, hiking, relationship and communication skills. The seminars and retreats I facilitated were called, Emotional Fitness™, and I offered private consultations for energy healing. It was during this time that the passed spirits of my clients' relatives began joining our sessions...a welcome surprise for everyone!

Welcome To My World

Suzane Northrop, Internationally-acclaimed medium, grief and bereavement expert, TV and radio host, and author of three books, also presented at Red Mountain Spa. It was wonderful to meet her and get to know her. And, I learned that she was actually Tara's teacher.

The night she was presenting, the person who was to introduce her had a conflict and asked me to do the introduction, which I was very happy to do. I went up to the designated function room early to be sure everything was ready. I opened the door and had to take a step back. Waiting there were so many spirits. It looked like 30 to 50...all very etheric and distinctly different from one another... waiting in suspension...just hanging out not touching the floor or the ceiling and spaced out evenly in silence. They knew Suzane would be there and they could get their messages heard. I took a quick look around the room and it had been set up. I excused myself and closed the door behind me. The thought went through my head that I could have talked to them, but I wasn't sure if that would be correct medium protocol. A short time later, I saw Suzane and told her my experience. She smiled knowingly and said, "Welcome to my world!"

About Spirits, the Spirit World and Messages Received

My experiences in the spirit dimension, as I have mentioned, have been heart-opening, healing and have supplied a basis of knowing the previously unknown as a deep unshakable knowing. I have found the spirit world consistent, congruent and judgeless and the messages refreshing and healing. I encourage you to venture into this realm if it draws you. Please note the resources and references at the end of this section.

Cautions about Working in This and Other Dimensions Energetically

I have been trained well to be safe travelling and working in spirit world and multiple and parallel dimensions. The law of "Where you put your attention becomes enlivened" is key here. It is important not to become fascinated or intrigued with dark entities, forces or energy.

We won't go into the description, beliefs or debates about what those are here. The bottom line is it is important to remember this is a sacred trek. Proper training, protocol, respect, assistance and focus are imperative. Pure intention and right use of all healing technologies with integrity and awareness must be implemented. Knowing your scope of knowledge, training and ability is, as always, important. One must stay at an intuitive, aware and reasonable state of gratitude, compassion and respect which is really no different from life in general.

The spirits I have had the honor of knowing have taught me they are actively supporting their loved ones on Earth. They wish to be in contact, communicate and assist and create better understanding of all realms. They have messages of healing, advice and remembering. They are limited by our lack of awareness of their presence and abilities. Following are three examples of spirit messages.

Mom on How to Solve the Problem

We were hiking in the wonderful Snow Canyon State Park in southern Utah. My business was really busy and I was frustrated about not being able to keep up with all I wanted to do. I was relating that to my husband and suddenly my mother, father, oldest brother and two uncles joined us...the problem is, they have all passed. They were consulting on what I could do to expand my business, do the training I wanted to and still see clients and do retreats. It was really humorous. Nothing had changed from when they were alive except that they seemed much more cohesive. As they talked, I related their ideas to my husband. He is used to this type of thing. They offered real and practical solutions which I took to heart and implemented. One idea was to call the local college computer studies department and post a job. They let me know they had to be on their way, and I sent them my love and gratitude. The next day I posted a job position at the college and found a delightful young woman who was unendingly helpful.

The Patchwork Quilt

A very dear friend of mine, John, called with a request. He knew I got messages from the spirit world and had just had a terrible tragedy in his family. His grandson, Jeff, who was 14 years old, had committed suicide. He was understandably deeply distraught and also very concerned for his daughter, who was totally devastated. He asked me if there was any way I could contact Jeff and find any kind of help at all to deal with what had happened. I didn't get an immediate connection and I told him I would do my best and get back to him.

The next day was a sunny, clear and cool morning, and the dogs were running ahead happily, and it was hard to imagine anyone could be sad. And then, as we turned the last bend to the way back home, the requested information came to me. A spirit like being of a young man who did not identify himself was showing me a small blue and white patchwork quilt with some patterns in the patches and trimmed in a dark sky blue. Then he "spoke" which is more telepathy than actual words and voice. "Please tell my mother and father, my brother and my grandpa that I love them very much and always will. And that there is nothing they did or said, or could have done or said that would have changed what happened. I am where I am supposed to be and it is part of a plan that is not comprehensible on Earth. Thank you for your help." I thanked him as he moved away from my sense of him, and I had arrived back at the house with the dogs.

The phone rang and it was John. He felt discouraged and wanted to know if I had found anything out. I told him about the information that was just given to me and he began to weep. He said that the patchwork quilt was Jeff's as a young child, and the family had draped his coffin with it in his memory. Tears welled up for me, too.

John was so grateful and was able to console his daughter and the rest of the family, and although the grief was still intense and painful, the message offered some resolution to all.

Signs and Signals and the Big Blue Dragonfly

Chandra chose to come to a retreat. One of the reasons she came was the passing of her father a short time before and she was

174

grieving his loss. I sensed her father's presence even before the retreat began, and that he was instrumental in leading her to the retreat. The spirits often come early.

It was Thursday and time for Chandra's private consultation with me. She is a young, beautiful woman inside and out. As she sat down, her father, whose name is Bob, appeared behind her on her right. He showed his earthly essence and was a handsome, very kind-hearted spirit and deeply loving soul.

I acknowledge his presence and described him to Chandra and she knew it was him right away. I gave her his message of deep love and caring and ask her to speak directly with him, and she did. It was a very touching reunion, and set the stage for her awareness of him as accessible and for further communication.

He mentioned he had been trying to contact her and asked if she had noticed. She said she felt his presence, but wasn't sure. I explained to her that spirits often use animals, birds, insects and electronic interference and other ways to get our attention. She took that in and it was as if a light went on.

She shared that her mom, Marge, and her dad loved Yellowstone Park and would spend a lot of time there. After Bob's death, Marge and Chandra went through the park and encountered a female Elk that would not take her eyes off of them for over an hour. Also, Marge's cell phone wouldn't work for two days "for no reason" and Chandra said that had to be him. Bob concurred. Later that day, Chandra told me as she left our consultation, a bunny rabbit ran in front of her and stopped and just sat there close to her. We worked on other issues she wanted to resolve, and Bob's spirit stood respectfully by. He stayed most of the retreat in love and support of Chandra.

In another private consultation about two to three years later, Chandra told me she was visiting her dad's grave and writing to him in her journal and a dragonfly landed on his gravestone. It didn't move for over twenty minutes and Chandra got basically nose to nose with it and said, "I know it's you Dad!" She asked if I thought it was him and Bob was again present and concurred.

Chandra and I discussed many issues and decisions she was facing, and worked on clarity and intention and released some emotions and beliefs that were in her way. We acknowledged Bob's presence, but he wasn't the main focus of our time together this time. We had a great session, and Chandra went on her way.

That afternoon, I was running some errands and placed my phone on the car seat. I heard it calling someone and picked it up as Chandra answered. I apologized and said it was a pocket call. But I knew it was more because she was not the last person I talked to. So I had the awareness her dad might have been involved with the call. Right then, a SUV pulled in front of me as I approached a red light. On the back window of the SUV was a huge blue dragonfly decal. It was about eighteen inches long. I got immediately that Chandra's dad wanted more acknowledgement and he desired to connect with her again and he confirmed that. It made me smile.

At that moment I was drawn to look at my dashboard and the milometer was at 47777. I've learned to pay attention to these signs and signals and called Chandra. I got her voicemail and relayed the story and message from Bob. Of course she was thrilled and sent me an email sharing her exhilaration. About three weeks later, I saw the same SUV and the giant blue dragonfly again in the lane next to me while driving across town. I took it as a "Thank you" from Bob.

A few months later, Chandra emailed that she and her mother went to Yellowstone Park to get away. With her permission, here is an excerpt from her message:

"As we travelled through the park we saw many animals; buffalo, elk, deer, antelope, and two black bears. However, on our way out of the park, we came across a mother grizzly and her little cub. We were up on a rise, looking through our binoculars in awe of the beautiful, playful animals. All of a sudden, at the same time we each started stuttering and going 'Hey, did you see?' We were jumping around. While we were both looking through our binoculars, the most brilliant blue dragonfly, as big as the moon, flew into both our views. We both began to cry and laugh at the same time. I felt the sign was for our continued healing. The similarity between the grizzly taking care of her young (mother/daughter) and that the dragonfly, appeared to help my mom understand that my dad is ok. It was a wonderful continuance of healing the grief, understanding of the spirit world and allowing the spirits to communicate. I am so thankful."

Becoming Official

I wanted to seek further credentials for the type of work I was now doing that evolved from my trainings and certifications in meditation, yoga, ayurveda, energy and intuitive work and had become a minister as well. I was facilitating my Emotional Fitness™ retreats, giving private consultations and had ventured out on my own and wanted to have official credentials for those kinds of activities since my work didn't require licensing.

Energy psychology is such a new area of healing, credentials had just started to become available. Thankfully, The Association for Comprehensive Energy Psychology had been organized and developed certification as a practitioner. I applied and completed the preparatory testing and requirements and booked to attend the first group certification at the ACEP Conference in Albuquerque. It was challenging, very informative and a perfect refinement of my skills and understanding.

I was a bit intimidated that licensed professionals, medical doctors, psychiatrists, psychologists, social workers, nurses and therapists made up most of our class. Even though I had majored in Speech and Hearing Sciences and minored in Psychology, I had not gone on to get my advanced degrees and had chosen the path of alternative and integrative medicine. Only three or four of us had come to the certification along those alternative pathways.

The first evening we were asked to stand up, introduce ourselves and give our backgrounds and reasons for seeking the certification. When it came to me, I stood up, still a little nervous, introduced myself and said that I was certified for meditation and ayurveda and used EFT and muscle testing and did retreats and seminars called Emotional Fitness and private consultations for healing and resolution of negative emotions. That was just fine but then the words, "I am also a spiritual intuitive and talk to dead people" just fell out of my mouth. Honestly, I was horrified and so was the very distinguished elder leader of the certification course. There was nothing else I could say or do at that time but say thank you and sit down and try to disappear. At the time I didn't know the benefits that statement would bring.

At lunch, three people, one M.D. one psychiatrist and one R.N., came up to me to relate a common thread of experience, interest and desire to increase the "spiritual" part of their practices. Another gentleman brought his wife over to me who was also intuitive and wanted to talk. I was so relieved and thankful and it was a perfect example of what happens when you speak your authentic truth even if some part of me didn't think I should have under the circumstances.

At the end of the group certification process, we were to select a mentor to monitor the completion of a certain number of hours of consultation work and our practice. Dr. Barbara Stone was one of the certification teachers and after reviewing the list of mentors and their work, I was immediately drawn to her and to her approaches. I found her to have a keen analytical mind and an equally keen spiritual acuity. A few months later, I received my ACEP certification, which has been especially beneficial in terms of learned skills, ethics guidelines support and common interests, and a community of colleagues I can consult and work with even if we are at a distance. That completion was only the beginning of a great expansion of the learning and healing adventure.

Soul Detective® Approach - Taking Energy Healing Work Higher, Deeper and Beyond Imagination

At that point, I chose to certify in Dr. Stone's healing work called, Soul Detective Work, and that process has opened door after door into learning and healing in ways I never even imagined. The Soul Detective approach promotes emotional well-being by using the tools from Energy Psychology to find and clear the origins of emotional disturbances. It fully integrates with my Emotional Fitness™ healing approach and I draw on the protocols often.

My personal healing experience with Soul Detective Work spans six years and has included my own certification as a Soul Detective Practitioner. Because of Dr. Stone's knowledge and fervent dedication to evolutionary healing, it has been and continues to be a leading edge and dynamic system of healing. It is extensive and expanding continually with ongoing support and consultation. It has brought a depth, breadth and higher meaning to my life, and the lives of my associates, colleagues and clients.

What I like about Soul Detective Work is that it is comprehensive, continually updated with new information and includes dependable methods and protocols. It is inclusive of the basic and expanded diagnostic and treatment tools of Energy Psychology and knows no limits of possibilities. Protocols include: Energy Assessment and Correction, Diagnostic Procedures, Customized Treatment Sequences, Past Life Trauma, Curses and Hexes, Soul Loss, Energetic Cords, Vows, Earthbound Spirits, Spirit Attachment, Obsessive Spirit Protocol, Ancestral Wounds, Releasing Dark and Detrimental Energy, Extraterrestrial Protocol, Archetypes and Soul Origin. The following are five examples of Soul Detective Work offered for a better understanding of how the inter-dimensional work resolves the origin of problems to help people live a happier, healthier life. Warning: These examples will more than likely create a belief gap unless you are familiar with this kind of work. Just keep an open mind and consider the, otherwise not possible, benefits of the healings process.

How a Past Life Healing Freed Me for This Life

I knew I was out of balance because I was feeling particularly insecure about my healing practice, getting certified for energy healing, and my writing. I was thinking things like "who do you think you are?" and "it's not worth all the work." Over time, this attitude about what I felt was my life work crept in repeatedly. Because there was a great deal of sadness attached to it, I decided to reach out to my mentor, Barbara Stone, originator of Soul Detective Work, and make an appointment for a session.

We determined that the origin of this problem was a past life trauma. Following the Soul Detective past life trauma protocol and using intuition, we discovered that I was Angelic Michelle, born along the coast of India in 127 AD. When we dropped into the lifetime, I was sitting in a grassy pasture on a hill overlooking the ocean, feeling happy and fearless. I was closely connected to Source, and my body felt radiant and etheric, even translucent. People came to me for the light, love, guidance and healing that my presence imparted.

The trauma began at the age of 13 when I sensed from Spirit that there would be a natural disaster coming to the island. I immediately began to try to warn the people of the village. They didn't want to hear what I said and thought I was tricking or betraying them. I was broken hearted and couldn't imagine why the people would feel that way. We paused here to do the tapping on the deep grief, shame and anxiety that I still held from that lifetime, that I had done something wrong and could not properly prepare the people of the village.

The tidal wave came. I was on the top of the hill where I had tried to persuade the people to come, but the wave was so monstrous it swept me and everyone else, including all the animals to our death and obliterated the island. Recalling this event triggered my long held fear of water, especially large waves, fear of not saying the right thing, or not saying or doing enough. This trauma and sudden death, the sadness and rage attached to that memory, had remained imprinted upon my soul and psyche. But, I realized there was nothing I could have done or said, or didn't do or say to save the people. This realization was very healing.

My soul's lesson was that a messenger of the Light was simply to impart Light in the form of possibilities and understanding, and that we do not have ultimate control of anything or anybody. The application of the healing of that time was to remember that if I feel frustration, self doubt and inadequacy and inability to control a situation, to let go and simply let the Light flow. After this healing, I was better able to be more accepting of all circumstances and remain simply a messenger of possibilities and understanding which I feel is my true purpose. I can have more fun in the surf too!

Making a Great Practice Better

A client I call Ethan is a forty-eight year old man who was referred to me by another client. He is a medical intuitive chiropractor and the referral was by his assistant. I know of this man and he is well respected in the community and considered a very good chiropractic doctor. He also carries herbs in his front office and other healing oils, Bach Flower essences and other supplements and healing substances. Although he prescribes various herbs and supplements, his assistant handles that side of the business entirely in terms of testing appropriateness and filling prescriptions.

He came to me because he said he didn't understand his "passive-aggressive" attitude towards stocking and prescribing the products he carries. He said he was guided to expand his business in this way and is puzzled by his "uncomfortableness" and "nervous reluctance" to use the products fully and freely with the appropriate clients.

He shared that he felt confident he was prescribing correctly, and he was getting good results for his patients, but he still had this discomfort around it, and was thinking of discontinuing that part of his practice. But, I thought I could possibly shed some light on the origins of the problem.

We did a centering and grounding exercise because he was visibly nervous and concerned. Following the Soul Detective protocol, we muscle tested for the origin of this problem and determined that the problem had original roots both in ancestral wounds and vows. Muscle testing further, we determined it was best to start with the ancestral wounds.

Following the protocol for ancestral wounds, we muscle tested that the ancestor was a female and was back four (4) generations on his Mother's side and so was his great, great grandmother. The client knew there were healers, doctors and herbalists on his mother's side. We did surrogate energy work for his great, great grandma to clear her trepidation, confusion, and her reluctance to serve, prescribe healing herbs.

At that point, the client shared that his mother came from a line of Native American "medicine" men/women. He said he knew that they had vowed not to reveal the healing secrets to anyone but the next of kin in line. He also had heard family stories about how some of them had been massacred for not doing what the "pioneers" had demanded. We then tested if his great, great grandmother had been massacred for this reason and it tested positive. We did the surrogate work (mainly EFT) for that traumatic death...she was just 23 at death. We also released her and Ethan from her vows not to tell anyone about the secret of healing as they were no longer applicable in this lifetime. We asked if she had crossed and all of her soul energy had not. She asked us to call her Marissa, and when we conversed with her, she gladly accepted the idea of returning to the "Nature Spirits" home with "The Great Spirit" and was carried up by the great "Eagle Spirit." Ethan had been told these names in family stories.

As is customary, we then offered multiplying the benefits for anyone else in the ancestral line and in the family, tribe and others concerned to be released from this energy dynamic.

We tested that the process was complete and Ethan was completely released from the influence of the ancestral wounds and vows. We then offered gratitude for spiritual help and healing opportunity and closed the session. Ethan demonstrated great relief and joy. He was so glad to have understanding about an issue that had plagued him daily for years.

In our two month follow-up call, Ethan shared that he has taken a personal and active role on all levels with his patients. His practice has expanded and he now speaks on herbal and essence healing with products from all over the world...something he had studied for years and had always been very knowledgeable about. As a side note, he married his assistant...☺who is now able to do what she was hired for in terms of accounting, receptionist and assistant for scheduling.

Vows to Keep and Vows to Break

Vows from previous lives that are still written on our Souls can cause unexplained problems in this life when they are no longer appropriate. Two cases were particularly applicable, and the irony of the circumstances of both situations is very interesting.

Meaningful Sex and Chastity

A client I call Dave, had suffered with a sex addiction for recent years and his wife, Diane, had found evidence of addiction to pornography on his computer. She was devastated with the betrayal. He was devastated with the reality of his actions and realized that, as in all addictions, he was looking for himself outside of himself.

I worked with both of them on the debilitating emotions generated by the circumstances to reduce the trauma and start picking up the pieces.

They decided he would go to a treatment center for several weeks. While he was in treatment, his wife struggled with ever taking him back and with the betrayal. They both did a lot of deep work, self inquiry and processing in an attempt to come to some sense of peace over this situation that had rocked their worlds.

They did come to some resolution and have continued trying to heal and reconstruct a viable relationship, partnership, and regain a meaningful sexual relationship. They were both struggling with that for their own reasons. Dave just didn't seem to be able to understand why it was so confusing and was crushed with guilt. In a private consultation with Dave, we muscle tested to find the origins of the deep guilt he just couldn't release. We found he had three vows of chastity from previous lifetimes as a clergyman. Of course, what a conflict! We released the vows and that action opened the doors for Dave and Diane to create an even better relationship than they had before. He replaced those vows with vows of loyalty to Diane.

Non-Profit Prosperity

Cynthia had created and expanded a very viable and needed non-profit organization that helps women all over the world be able to get proper health care, particularly in the areas of women's issues and pregnancy and childbirth. Cynthia had collaborated with many doctors and health organizations and the organization was able to reach more and more women this way. The problem was that it was getting more and more difficult to obtain the necessary donations to take care of all the women that desperately needed this medical help.

We muscle tested for the origin of lack of prosperity, abundance and flow of finances and found she had taken vows of poverty from previous lifetimes in ecclesiastical orders that required these vows. We also realized that the inherent nature of the title, "non-profit" intimates "no profit" and was a limiting concept. We removed the vows and Cynthia felt a great sense of relief and freedom. We replaced the vows with a vow of abundance and prosperity as a sacred path. We will do a two month follow-up and I fully expect the lack of abundance will be a thing of the past.

How Alternate Beginnings Help Create Alternate Endings

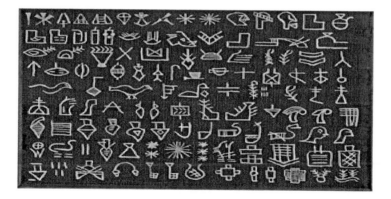

The Sumerian alphabets have always held some unexplained attraction for me. The stories of the Sumer and the Anunnaki Gods from the planet Neibiru and the ancient archeological theories about Sumer and extra terrestrials inhabiting earth have been fascinating as well. I was aware that there was a lot of collaboration and agreement about unexplained archeological sites among writers, ancient archeological theorists and historians about the very tall, stately alien beings, the Anunnaki. They were believed to be known as aggressive and controlling and possibly connected to certain aberrations in the human body attributed to the developing of a species of slaves by altering DNA, gene splicing and fusing vertebrae. An underlying motivation was that they needed and wanted the Earth's gold for their survival.

That was a belief gap I wasn't motivated to go into, but I was kept informed through the multidimensional network of friends and ET specialists. Also, I would happen to catch the discussion on specials on the History Channel and note occasional references to Zecharia Sitchin, author and researcher of extensive detailed writing regarding the extensive Sumerian Tablets and the Anunnaki. Now that I am writing about it, I realize it has been a constant inflow of bits of information over time.

I had never thought much about the other historical scenarios and was neutral about ET's and aliens. Certainly, biblical and archeological and evolutionary accounts of human and earthly evolution and history never really added up for me. I neither believed nor disbelieved they existed and/or inhabited the earth at some point, or are present now. I had seen odd things in the sky and always wondered about crop circles, but to my knowledge, I had never had an ET encounter. It was always just a passing event that caught my attention and contemplation about possible alternative beginnings on Earth and ET sightings...until...

Updates to the Soul Detective Protocols that included detrimental energies and ET's and information about the Anunnaki Gods began to show-up in my inbox. Also, on our Soul Detective conference calls, I was able to hear case studies using the latest protocols. As I learned more and realized the far reaching opportunities for new understanding and healing, I began to bridge the belief gap and engage in thinking about the alternate possibilities to explain the origins of issues in this life. As always, I also began to use the new protocols in my private consultations. The depth and breadth of healing was unmistakable. It prompted me to complete the requirements of my Soul Detective Certification and to host Levels I, II, and III Soul Detective trainings for professionals with Dr. Stone to help spread the word and to refresh and renew my knowledge and skills...And then...

Communication with the Anunnaki

It was one of the last days of the certification. That day we were reviewing the latest and most advanced healing protocols, and we were testing for detrimental energies and possible ET interference. I was already astounded at the massive information, learning, healing and practice we had already covered, and now felt very interested in advancing my understanding about the information that was newer for me. Little did I know it was going to be an up front and personal experience. **Warning: This will definitely produce a belief gap.**

Implementing the protocol for detrimental energies and/or ET interference, Barbara skillfully muscle tested to determine if there were any interference patterns in my field. There were 19! Two were beneficial, seven detrimental and ten were neutral. We methodically identified them and resolved them one by one. They ranged from energy interference of elemental forms asking for more understanding and respect, to energetic forms to cloud my intuition and keep shame and hopelessness in my field, to attempts to disintegrate my heart energy, to monitor my travels and activities possibly for their research, and to usurp some of the flow of consciousness from me.

The most astounding form of control or interference was a barely discernible clear barrier of detrimental energy in front of me for as far as I could see or imagine. When I asked why this was here, the answer was "to keep me from moving forward, keep me from accessing the future or other dimensions, and monitor my speed" like a governor on a car. At that moment, three figures came into my mind's view. They were undeniably Anunnaki from all the descriptions I had ever seen or heard, and were very tall, Egyptian like stately figures standing in a triangle with what appeared to be a young female in front. I felt an immediate kinship with them which was very puzzling to me. The young female spoke her name, "I am Ansa," and then said, "Too many people are moving too fast for us. We decided to control everyone indiscriminately. We realize now that was not the right thing to do."

I was shocked as these Anunnaki were apologizing and speaking to me. Ansa continued, "We felt pushed back and threatened. Angels came to us and explained that it is true some people need to be stopped, but not all. They needed us to realize there are forces that can align, co-create and co-exist. We want to see if that is possible."

She introduced her father behind her on her right, Anki, and her mother behind her on her left, Ash. They didn't move or speak. Anza continued communicating their collective thought. They began dissolving or melting the barrier in front of me. They explained that they simply change the frequency to do that. The barrier appeared to morph and curl down forming a sort of doorway and corridor.

Still unclear as to who needs to be stopped and who doesn't, they explained they believe they have the true view of the universe and that there are too many people on Planet Earth that are destructive. Their criteria for peace are changing as they are considering the possibilities for a peaceful coexistence. Anza said, "We now are willing to allow the angels to join our council meetings and some earthlings as well. We didn't ever know any way to survive except by controlling everything. Thank you for listening." They then bowed ever so slightly lowering their eyes and disappeared into the background. I didn't want them to leave.

As we finished the healing session, we found that the change in the frequency of the barrier resolved the remaining interferences. As we finished the muscle testing to be sure all was complete, I still had my eyes closed, and Sumerian symbols filled my screen of inner vision.

I must say that this was one of the most profound healing sessions I have experienced. It was an opening to never discounting energy and information coming in to your awareness. As I look back at my history of getting acquainted with the dimensional world, I can see the path that led to this experience. Since the healing session, I have been more focused, have experienced more lateral and out of the box thinking, and my energy level and adventurous spirit have expanded, and I have had no bouts with frustration and feelings of hopelessness. I am grateful and looking forward to more encounters with the other-dimensional beings.

Multidimensional Healing Resource Guide:

Second Chance: Messages from the Afterlife, Everything Happens for a Reason: Love, Free Will & Lessons of the Soul, A Medium's Cookbook: Recipes for the Soul, by Suzane Northrop

www.SuzaneNorthrop.com

Invisible Roots: How Healing Past Life Trauma Can Liberate Your Present, by Barbara Stone, Ph.D.

Transforming Fear into Gold:

How Facing What Frightens You the Most Can Heal and Light up Your Hear, by Barbara Stone, Ph. D

When Time Began: Book V of the Earth Chronicles, by Zecharia Sitchin

www.history.com/ancient-aliens

www.souldetective.net

www.mergingrivers.com

Section Six

An Introduction to Three Comprehensive Healing Systems to Support and Sustain Your Healing Path and Joyous Life

Ayurveda

An ancient, eloquent and elegant complex and comprehensive world healing system, and the East Indian traditional system of medicine, Ayurveda (pronounced Aa-yer-vay-da) is called the science of life or longevity.

I was introduced to Ayurveda through Dr. Deepak Chopra's books which I passionately read and collected. I found the information like going home because it follows the natural way I was brought up. It is based on the universal laws and is an intricate, multi-layered science. It is a complex detailed system incorporating all levels of existence and it takes many years to become an Ayurvedic doctor and/or practitioner. As I fell in love with Ayurveda, the universe answered my desires to learn and experience more about it. I had the great fortune to study with Drs. Chopra and Simon and become an Ayurvedic instructor.

The great thing about Ayurveda is that just a little basic knowledge and understanding and experience of the healing system can be significantly beneficial to your health, well-being and sense of personal empowerment. The purpose of this chapter is to provide you with an introduction of Ayurveda with knowledge and understanding and awareness that will raise your level of health and well-being, and give you a more accurate image of your true identity making your choice points more successful.

Ayurveda was first known through a spiritual tradition of a universal religion for which healers from over the world would gather in India and share their knowledge. It has a fascinating origin and history. It is also purported that the vast knowledge was intuited during meditation and directly passed down from God to Angels, and then to humans through direct cognition and divine revelation. The whole subject of how all medical knowledge, treatments and therapies have come into existence is fascinating in itself. In any case, it is a complete and comprehensive scientific system based on basic universal field premises, and includes the following eight branches:

1. Internal Medicine (Mind and Body and the Soul) - Health is not the absence of disease, but the optimum flow and balance of biological humors and life energy.
   a. Psychosomatic Theory – An imbalanced mind can create illness and a healthy mind is instrumental in healing disease.

b. Seven Body/Mind Constitutions Vata/Air, Pitta/Fire, Kapha/ Water, Vata/Pitta, Vata/Kapha, Pitta/Kapha, Tridoshic

c. Finding the origin of illness through the six developmental stages of illness: aggravation (irritability and decreased function), accumulation (inflammation), overflow, relocation, buildup in a new site, manifestation into a recognizable disease.

d. Comprehensive Ayurvedic Therapies: Herbology, Nutrition, Meditation, Pranayam, Pancha Karma, Abhyanga, Aromatherapy, Hatha Yoga Therapy, Daily Routine, Head Massage, Sound Therapy: Mantras, Chakras, Music, Chanting, Color, Gem, Ash Therapies, Lifestyle Counseling and Exercise, Psychology, Ethics, and Spiritual Counseling, Numerology, Astrology

2. Ears, Nose and Throat - Includes all eye, ear, nose and throat diseases, disorders.

3. Toxicology – Keys to recognizing pollution, toxins and epidemics and their antidotes.

4. Pediatrics – Prenatal and postnatal care of baby and mother, including methods of conception; choosing the child's gender, intelligence and constitution; childhood diseases and midwifery.

5. Surgery – All types of sophisticated methods of surgery.

6. Psychiatry - Diseases of the mind (including demonic possession). Herbs, diet, yoga therapy, pranayam, chanting are included in the therapies.

7. Aphrodisiacs – Deals with infertility and also for spiritual development to transmute sexual energy into spiritual energy.

8. Rejuvenation – Prevention and longevity are the focus of this branch, as well as ethics and virtuous living.

The practice of Ayurvedic knowledge opens the possibility for better health through higher awareness, clearer thoughts, interpretations, perceptions and consequently, best choices.

The universal premises of Ayurveda we will explore are these:

• All life is innately self-healing

• We are all one and individually unique and complete microcosms or the macrocosm of existence

• Everything is made of the same universal elements or energies – Ether, Air, Fire, Water and Earth

- We all have a unique mind/body constitution made up of the elemental energies. And, for optimum potentiality, these elements must be in appropriate balance
- Life is an expression of the field of consciousness which is our basic nature, and consciousness is unbounded.
- Exploring the field of consciousness is the basis of healing and the basic forms of exploration are study, meditation, pranayam and yoga

Four Main Thrusts of Ayurvedic Living

We will explore four of the many areas of Ayurvedic teachings in the effort to supply information and awareness that will add to knowledgeable self realization and self-care, and assist with the many choice points we face daily regarding self-knowledge, personal choice, nutrition and well-being. They include, mind/body composition, secrets of dynamic balance, nutrition and purification and daily routine.

Your Individual Mind/Body Composition

On the next page is a very brief mind/body quiz you can complete to get an idea of your basic Doshic Constitution makeup. Although this quiz is basically reliable, it is only designed and intended to give a working indication of your Doshic makeup. If you were to have a complete Ayurvedic assessment from an Ayurvedic doctor or practitioner, it would entail a full examination and many questions and evaluations incorporating the many layers of considerations regarding your health and well-being.

Mind/Body Constitution Doshic Constitution Quiz

Please mark the selection that best describes you most of the time, and total each column where indicated. We all have all the elements air, fire, water, earth and ether in our mind/body makeup. There is most often a predominant element and a second dominant one. There are seven categorizations: As an example, if you had five Air/Vata selections and three Fire/Pita selections and two Earth/Kapha selections, your mind/body constitution would be referred to as Air/Vata/Fire/Pitta. If you have equal numbers of selections for all three, your constitution would be referred to as TriDoshic. If you have questions, refer to the detailed chart below the quiz to help you with clarity about the qualities that best describe you and your unique mind/body constitution.

Characteristic	Air/Vata	Fire/Pitta	Earth/Kapha
Frame	I am thin, lanky, and slender with prominent joints and thin muscles.	I have a medium symmetrical build with good muscle development.	I have a large, round or stocky build. My frame is broad, stout or thick.
Weight	Low - I may forget to eat or have a tendency to lose weight.	Moderate - It is easy for me to loose or gain weight if I put my mind to it.	Heavy - I gain weight easily and have difficulty loosing it.
Eyes	My eyes are small and active.	I have a penetrating gaze.	I have large pleasant eyes.
Complexion	My skin is dry, rough or thin.	My skin is warm, reddish in color and prone to irritation.	My skin is, thick, moist and smooth.
Hair	My hair is dry, brittle or frizzy.	My hair is fine with a tendency towards early thinning or graying.	I have abundant, thick and oily hair.
Joints	My joints are thin and prominent and have a tendency to crack.	My joints are loose and flexible.	My joints are large, well-knit and padded.
Sleep Pattern	I am a light sleeper with a tendency to awaken easily.	I am a moderately sound sleeper, usually needing less than eight hours to feel rested.	My sleep is deep and long. I tend to awaken slowly in the morning.
Body Temperature	My hands and feet are usually cold and I prefer warm environments.	I am usually warm, regardless of the season, and prefer cooler environments.	I am adaptable to most temperatures but do not like cold, wet days.
Temperament	I am lively and enthusiastic by nature. I like to change.	I am purposeful and intense. I like to convince.	I am easy-going and accepting. I like to support.
Under Stress...	I become anxious and/or worried.	I become irritable and/or aggressive.	I become withdrawn and/or reclusive.
Totals	Air/Vata: _____	Fire/Pitta: _____	Earth/Kapha: _____

Circle your constitution based on your scores.
1. Air/Vata   4. Air/Vata-Fire/Pitta   7. TriDoshic
2. Fire/Pitta,   5. Air/Vata-Earth/Kapha
3. Earth/Kapha.   6. Fire/Pitta-Earth/Kapha

Doshic Qualities

Air/Vata Expansion and Movement	Fire/Pitta Chemical Transformation	Earth/Kapha Structure and Lubrication
Qualities Cold, Light, Dry, Irregular, Rough, Mobile, Quick, Changeable	Qualities Hot, Light, Intense, Penetrating, Pungent, Sharp, Acidic	Qualities Cold, Heavy, Solid, Stable, Smooth, Slow
Source of Thinking, Neuromuscular Activity, Respiration, Circulation, Digestive Movement	Source of Mental Discrimination, Visual Perception, Digestion and Metabolism / Skin Complexion, Temperature Regulation	Source of Supporting and nourishing the nervous system, Lubricating the digestive tract, the joints, the respiratory tract, and Regulating water and fat
Prominent Constitution Preponderance of the Air Principle and possess attributes that resemble the wind	Prominent Constitution Predominance of the Fire Principle and have a fiery nature that manifests in both body and mind	Prominent Constitution An abundance of Earth Principle and typically grounded and steady, remaining unruffled by and sometimes resistant to change
Mind Body Characteristics Thin and light build; active, open to change; variable routine; delicate appetite and digestion	Mind Body Characteristics Medium build; strong digestion, thinning or gray hair; warm body temperature; perspires easily; sleeps soundly for short periods of time; strong sex drive	Mind Body Characteristics Heavyset; smooth skin; thick hair; sweet face; deep sound sleep; slow moving; regular digestion; gains weight easily and has difficulty losing it; good stamina; slow and easy sex drive; process-oriented
Temperament Welcome new experiences; doesn't like routine; is a lively conversationalist; spends money easily	Temperament Sharp intellect; discriminating; direct; precise; stays close to routine; courageous; good teacher/speaker; spends money on luxury items	Temperament Easy going and patient; thoughtful; stable; content; devoted; loving; comfortable with routine; saves money
In Balance Energetic; creative; adaptable, shows initiative; good communicator	In Balance Bright; warm; good decision-maker; strong digestion	In Balance Steady; consistent; loyal; strong; supportive
Out of Balance Shows mental agitation, anxiety, worry, inconsistency, insomnia, gas and bloating, constipation Stress Response: "What did I do wrong?"	Out of Balance Angry; irritable; excessively critical or harsh; judgmental, aggressive; intimidating; skin rashes; burning sensations, indigestion Stress Response: "What did you do wrong?"	Out of Balance Dull; inert; needy; attached; congested; overweight; overly-protective Stress Response: "I don't want to deal with it."

Creating and Maintaining Dynamic Balance

The concept of balancing in Ayurveda is different from our normal way of looking at balancing. It doesn't mean that you seek to make each element equal with the other. It does mean if you are feeling out of balance, there is too much of an element accumulated in the mind, body and environment. Air/Vata out of balance is too much air and symptoms are feeling ungrounded and unable to focus, moving too fast. A common emotion is anxiety. Fire/Pitta out of balance is too much fire and symptoms are irritation and aggressive feelings or actions. Earth/Kapha out of balance is too much earth and symptoms of sluggishness, congestion or dullness.

To balance the focus is not on "getting rid" of the excess, it is on adding a balancing element.

For example, for too much air, bring in stability and earth qualities; for too much fire, bring in more space and coolness; for too much Earth, bring in movement and circulation. So it is an attitude of balancing with adding qualities. The chart below groups balancing choices into the Six Tastes. The goal of the Six Tastes is to balance and include all every day.

The Six Tastes and Ayurvedic Balancing

We can't "get rid of" anything. We must either seek or avoid the foods, habits and experience that will balance whatever we have too much of or are deficient in. Our Mind/Body Opposites are cures for opposites. Review the charts on the next pages to familiarize and understand the Ayurvedic balancing premise.

The Basic Components of Balancing
The Six Tastes (relate to food, people, activity, experience and environment)

Dosha	Element	Taste/Function	Examples
Air/Vata	Ether	Astringent-Drying, Compacts System	Beans, tea, apples, pomegranates, cauliflower, dark leafy greens (tannins)
	Air	Bitter-Anti-inflammatory, Detoxifying	Green, leafy vegetables, eggplant, radishes celery, sprouts, beets, (alkaloids, glycosides)
Fire/Pitta	Fire	Pungent-Stimulates Digestion, Clears Congestion	Hot peppers, salsa, ginger, radishes, mustard, cloves, horseradish (essential oils)
	Water	Salty-Mildly Laxative/Sedative, Promotes Digestion	Salt, sauces, salted meats and fish (mineral salt)
Earth/ Kapha	Earth	Sour-Improves Appetite & Digestion, Promotes Digestion	Citrus fruits, yogurt, cheese, tomatoes, salad dressings, pickles, vinegar (organic acids)
		Sweet-Most Nutritive, Builds Body Tissue	Sugar, honey, milk, butter, rice, breads, pastas, meats, (carbohydrates, fats, proteins)

Further Considerations in Balancing the Doshas

Consideration	Air/Vata	Fire/Pitta	Earth/Kapha
Temperatures	Keep warm Avoid extreme cold	Avoid excessive heat, steam	Avoid excessive humidity
Mood	Keep calm	Cultivate compassion	Seek stimulation
Foods	Avoid cold, frozen or raw foods Eat warm cooked foods/ spices	Avoid excessive oil Eat cool, raw non-spicy foods	Avoid fatty, oily foods Avoid iced food or drinks Eat light, dry food
Tastes	Favor sweet, sour, salty	Favor sweet, bitter, astringent	Favor bitter, astringent, pungent
Environment	Favor moist, warm, calm	Favor cool, fluid, orderly	Favor warm, dry active
Routine	Keep a regular routine	Be flexible and adapt routine	Keep a spacious routine
Rest	Get plenty of rest	Adequate rest	No daytime naps
Oil Massage	Sesame, almond	Coconut, sesame	Sesame, eucalyptus
Exercise	Swim, dance, weight train	Exercise during cool hours Non-competitive sports	Get plenty of vigorous exercise

Elemental Vibrational Balance and Imbalance

The interrelated nature and dynamic balance of the body mind and emotions

Dosha Function	Element	Taste	Emotion/ Ama Excess	Emotion/Ojas Moderation
Tissue Growth Development	Earth/Water	Sweet	Attachment Clingy	Satisfaction Stable
Kapha				
Mineral and Water Balance	Fire/Water	Sour	Greed Hedonism	Zest Visionary
Maintain Acidity and Thrist	Earth/Fire	Salty	Envy Resentment	Adventurous Daring
Pitta				
Metabolism Appetite Digestion	Fire/Air	Pungent	Hatred Rage	Extroverted Gregarious
Detoxification/Depleting	Air/Space	Bitter	Grief Pessimism	Desire to change Optimism
Vata				
Firmness of Tissue	Air/Earth	Astringent	Fear Insecurity	Introspection Self Esteem

Purification and Nutrition

Ayurveda is very clear about the need for purification and proper nutrition as a way of life and, as is true of all Ayurvedic practices, there are volumes of information about the various methods and therapies. It is an ongoing process of constant detoxification, purification and renewal, and of diligently reducing *Ama* (toxins) and creating *Ojas* (vigor/essential life energy). This is done with the whole organism and its environment in mind, incorporating harmony with natural cycles, getting proper nutrition and nurturing, treating food as medicine, detoxification, purification and daily routine. This applies to all levels of being: physical, emotional, mental, spiritual and environmental. Ayurvedic remedies are abundant throughout the Ayurvedic texts. These methods serve as preventative measures and in circumstances of treating and recovering balance from illness. The following list, recipe and eating philosophy are offered as samples for your learning awareness of the innumerable and comprehensive Ayurvedic detoxification, purification and rejuvenating methods.

Purification Guidelines Regarding Detoxification and Renewal

Ayurveda never says "never"...You will hear "favor" and "avoid" in reference to personal choice and healing recommendations. Remember that an Ayurvedic path is an informed lifestyle and is about personal knowledge, awareness and experience.

For Purification, Avoid the Following Foods:
<u>Ama (Toxin) Increasing Foods</u>
    Sweet Fruits
    Potatoes, mushrooms, carrot juice (too sweet alone)
    Breads, pastries, white flour
    All other beans not found on the next list
    Nuts and other seeds
    Meat, fish, poultry, eggs, lard
    Dairy
    Oils
    Sugars
    Salt
    Cold liquids, coffee

To Aide in the Reduction of Ama, Favor These Foods
<u>Āma Reducing Foods</u>
    Lemon, lime, grapefruit, pomegranate, cranberry
    Steamed vegetables for Vata and Kapha
    Raw vegetables for Pitta
    Whole grains (oats and wheat in moderation)
    Kichari
    Mung beans
    Pumpkin seeds moderately
    Acidophilus, yogurt, water
    Ghee (moderation), mustard, flax oils
    Raw honey
    Spices
    Warm liquids (teas)

Ayurvedic All Dosha Cleansing Tea

This is a purification tea best taken on an empty stomach. (Please note adaptations for individual Doshas). Simmer fresh cleaned and cut ginger in purified water. Add fresh lemon juice and pure honey as needed.

Vata/Air imbalance - use more honey and more lemon
Pitta/Fire imbalance - use more honey and less ginger
Kapha/Earth imbalance - use less honey and more ginger
Enjoy!

Ayurvedic Wisdom Eating

Food is energy. Eat only the energy you wish to be
Eat when you are hungry on an empty stomach
Feel Grace—the appreciation for the energy of the food
Eating is an intimate act, be reverent
Consider the source and preparation with gratitude
Choose your food as if you love yourself
Eat to balance
Eat only until you are not quite full
Eat your main meal in the middle of the day
Do not eat when upset (an angry person can turn the nectar of
the gods into poison)
When you are upset, drink water, breathe, and meditate
Eat in a settled atmosphere
Always sit down to eat
Avoid ice-cold drinks with food
Eat or Talk
Be aware of the pace you eat...savor
Sip warm water or herbal tea with meals
Eat a variety of tastes and colors of food
Avoid leftovers
Sit quietly for a few minutes or take a relaxing walk after you eat

Daily Routine

Ayurveda is based on the premise that natural reoccurring or activity and rest cycles dictate and demonstrate the natural processes of all life. Since we are expressions of nature, the natural cycles influence our mental, emotional and physical being on many levels. Entraining with the natural cycles results in conscious balance and optimum health and well-being. The current epidemic of stress and the symptoms of stress from constant activity on all levels 24/7, is a symptom in imbalance of the activity and rest cycle. The Ayurvedic approach is to make efforts to reconnect to the natural cycles to correct the imbalance. The cycles include the twenty-four hour Circadian Rhythms, the 12-month Seasonal Rhythms, the monthly lunar cycles and the gravitational Tidal Rhythms.

Daily routine is highly revered and the following is a suggested ideal daily routine of activities that are most supported by the natural cycles in play each day. Of course, you ultimately need to experiment and design your own daily routine based on your individual needs, mind/body make up, activities and environment. In addition to a daily cycle, Ayurvidic wisdom prescribes awareness of the lunar and tidal rhythms, as well as purification and change in diet to balance seasonal changes at the equinox and solstice times of year.

Morning

- Awaken before dawn without an alarm clock
- Brush your teeth, clean your tongue and massage your gums
- Drink a glass of warm water
- Empty your bowels and bladder
- Massage your body with warm oil (important aspect of the daily routine that provides a stable influence all year long. Oils recommended are almond and sesame for Air/Vata; coconut, sunflower, olive for Fire/Pitta; sunflower, mustard, almond for Earth/Kapha)
- Bathe or shower (recommended hydrotherapy/ cold shower to stimulate blood to the skin)
- Perform flexibility exercises around sunrise (yoga, meditation, spiritual practice)
- Eat breakfast with awareness
- Perform your morning work and/or activity

Mid-day

- Eat lunch: noon to 1:00 pm (largest meal of the day)
- Sit quietly for five minutes after eating
- Walk five to fifteen minutes to aid digestion
- Perform your afternoon work and activity
- Meditate around sunset

Evening

- Eat dinner: 6:00 to 7:00 P.M. (light to moderate)
- Sit quietly for five minutes after eating
- Walk five to fifteen minutes to aid digestion
- Attempt to be in bed with the lights off by 10:30 P.M

For further study and application of the empowering Ayurvedic system of healing, please note the resources below.

Ayurveda Resource Guide for Further Study:

Ayurvedic Healing – A Comprehensive Guide, by David Frawley
Ayurveda, The Science of Self Healing – A Practical Guide, by Vasant Lad
The Complete Book of Ayurvedic Home Remedies, by Vasant Lad
Perfect Health – The Complete Mind/Body Guide, by Deepak Chopra, M.D.
Creating Health – How to Wake Up the Bodies Intelligence, by Deepak Chopra, M.D.
The Wisdom of Healing, by David Simon, M.D.
The Ayurveda Encyclopedia – Natural Secrets to Healing, Prevention, and Longevity, by Swami Sada Shiva Tirtha
www.chopracenter.com
www.mergingrivers.com

Kundalini Yoga and Meditation – Technology for the Soul

I will tell you about yoga in very simple terms: The human mind is potentially infinite and creative. But in practical reality, it is limited. So a technical knowhow is required through which one can expand one's mind to bring about the equilibrium that enables one to control one's physical structure and experience one's infinite self.

-Yogi Bhajan, Ph.D.

It was 1968 and it was raining. My husband, Hub and I had just moved to Portland, Oregon for a new job opportunity with Heath Candy Company in the new business field of school fundraising. I was assisting him as he developed his new five-state territory. I also chose to go back to school and take some post graduate classes in speech and hearing therapy and psychology at Portland State University. I had also registered for a continuing education yoga class at the high school near our home.

The yoga class was every Wednesday evening from 7:00 to 9:00 P.M. for six weeks. It was taught by a very distinguished man from India who wore a turban and white clothing whose name I couldn't pronounce and can't remember. I was very intrigued and loved the class. I didn't know what kind of yoga it was and didn't even really know there were different kinds of yoga. In those days, yoga classes were rare in the west, and "yoga was yoga."

I was very busy with setting up our new home, helping Hub, and going to school. By Wednesdays at 7:00 P.M., I was tired and stressed and normally would not want to go anywhere. I went to the class anyway because I knew how refreshed, relaxed and renewed I would feel by the end of class. I looked forward to it every week and the six weeks went by quickly. I fully intended to sign up for the next semester's class, but was told the teacher had returned to India and no yoga was being offered. I was disappointed and didn't know at that time that I would not find a class like that again for almost thirty years.

It was 2006 and it was sunny. I had been part of the guest education staff for Red Mountain Resort in Ivins, Utah for four years now. I was leaving the fitness building after a meditation class I was teaching, and as I walked down the hallway by fitness studio one and looked in the open door. The yoga teacher dressed in white and wearing a turban-like head covering, waved me in and said, "Come to the class. Come on, why not?" Well, I had the right clothes on and I couldn't think of a reason why not, so I joined the class.

The teacher's name was Benja. She was a very skillful teacher and all of the 1968 experiences of the yoga class began to stream through me and I knew I had found the yoga I had been looking for. Two weeks later, my friend and colleague, Ann, the fitness director, waved a brochure at me down that same hallway and said, "Hey, do you want to do this teacher training for Kundalini Yoga?" I said, "Sure, why not." and that was the beginning of the most integrating and transformational training I have ever done.

Many people discover Kundalini Yoga in similar sudden ways. The technology speaks to all that we are, and can be easily intuited and instantly enjoyed. A previous belief about Marshal Arts and yoga practice is that it took many years to be a master and receive the true benefits and took total devotion of one's life. Perhaps it is true that it still takes time to be a master, however, Kundalini practice can be noticeably effective in as little as three minutes of practice and is designed to practice along with whatever lifestyle responsibilities you may have. Yogi Bhajan, who brought this yoga to the west in the late 60's, called Kundalini Yoga and Meditation a "householders yoga" for that reason. He was not seeking followers. He was teaching teachers to teach to spread the word about the healing technology of Kundalini Yoga. The technology was originally for only royalty and other privileged persons, and is now available to anyone. It is an inclusive system of healing and an internationally trained and taught technology of self awareness and enlightenment in all different cultures and societies.

We are fortunate that the people who surrounded him and his teachings had the foresight to film and record his vast body of teachings he offered daily over the more than forty years he served as the Master Teacher of Kundalini in the western world. We enjoy archives of information to draw from for teachings for a lifetime full of learning regarding all aspects of life.

What is Kundalini Yoga and What Does It Offer?

Kundalini means "pure awareness." It is the energy of pure consciousness and normally lies dormant in our lower chakras. With the process of knowledge, awareness and experience leading to enlightenment, the Kundalini energy rises into the upper chakras and throughout our field of energy. This process and experience allows us to perceive the etheric reality we really are, one of harmony, peace and purpose. The caduceus symbol of two snakes entwined is often used to show the finite and infinite nature and understanding rising up the chakras.

Kundalini Yoga offers a lifestyle that seeks optimum health and well-being on all levels and extraordinary human excellence. It includes many forms of yoga as a comprehensive technology based on the science of how energy moves. It is called a Raj yoga, king of yoga, because it has kept the incorporation of all aspects of the yoga practice fundamentals. It also includes all aspects of the six philosophies of yoga, Patanjalies eight limbs of yoga, and Sutras. Kundalini Yoga and meditation techniques have been called the owner's manual for human consciousness.

Kundalini yoga sets (kriyas) and meditations are prescriptive. In other words, they have specific technique and intent. For example, there are sets to be disease free, for spiritual elevation, to strengthen the nervous system, to clear and tone the chakras, to expand communication, to open the heart, to strengthen the immune system. There are literally thousands of kriyas and meditations. The teacher will choose one according to what he/she feels is needed for any specific class.

This Yoga is a known formula for happiness
and the experience of your human excellence

- Yogi Bhajan, Ph.D.

Known Benefits of the Practice of the Kundalini Yoga and Meditation Technology

- Balances the entire human energy field
- Detoxifies the glandular system
- Strengthens the nervous system

- Cleanses the subconscious
- Calms and develops the mind
- Realigns and strengthens the body
- Releases blocks, negativity and fear
- Elevates the spirit
- Tones the physical body from the inside out
- Resolves addiction and compulsion
- Develops pure conscious awareness
- Lifts your pure awareness and sense of divinity to its potential

Components of the Practice of Kundalini Yoga

- Breath (Pranayam)
- Sound/Vibration/Chanting (Mantras & Music)
- Body Movement (Asanas)
- Hand and Eye Positions (Mudras)
- Moving, Mantra and Silent Meditations
- Life Teachings
- Deep Relaxation

Kundalini Teachings

Kundalini Yoga and Meditation practice includes addressing all areas of life.

- Awakening Consciousness
- Pranayam
- Kriyas
- Relaxation
- The Mind
- Meditation
- Spiritual Practice
- Yogic Anatomy
- Yogic Philosophy
- Spiritual Development
- Humanology, including life cycles, relationship, excellence as a man or a woman, parenting, death, prosperity, happiness, integrity, communication, purpose
- Yogic Lifestyle
- Yogic Diet

Keeping Your Kundalini Experience Safe

Kundalini Yoga is a powerful transformational technology an inherently safe, natural practice. As in all powerful things, if they are used incorrectly, mindlessly or carelessly, the results can be undesirable. Kundalini classes are taught in a way that is non-competitive and to create a sacred and safe space for your personal experience. Anyone who can breathe can do Kundalini Yoga because it is taught energetically and does not require any specific background or abilities. Please take note and follow the guidelines below when learning and practicing Kundalini Yoga and Meditation to insure your experience is blissfully transformative with grace and ease as it is intended to be. Self responsibility is one of the teachings.

- Learn only from an Internationally Certified Kundalini Teacher who is certified in Kundalini Yoga and Meditation as taught by Yogi Bhajan, Ph.D.
- Do not practice Kundalini Yoga and Meditation under the influence of drugs, alcohol or other mind-altering drugs. In the case of prescribed psychotropic drugs, ask your doctor's permission.
- Practice regularly, challenge yourself, but do not push yourself past your comfortable limits.

Stay hydrated and listen closely to your body and to the teacher's guidance. Sat Nam

International Kundalini Yoga Class Structure

You have only one friend, your own conscious awareness and discipline. This is what will protect you and keep you strong. Merge with the universe and enjoy.

- Yogi Bhajan, Ph.D.

Kundalini classes will vary from instructor to instructor, and depending on the intention of the class. They will range from meditative to physically vigorous and every combination in between. They will never be the same, but they will always include the following:

- **Tune in Mantra – Ong Namo Guru Dev Namo**
  Tuning the individual field frequency to the universal field frequency of information, knowledge and energy

- **Pranayam and Warm Up If Needed**
  Waking up the body and mind to release stress, receive the experiential learning and balancing

- **Kriya, Lesson, and Set**
  A prescriptive set of movements, mantras, pranayam to accomplish the intention of the class to activate, balance and elevate the entire human field

- **Deep Relaxation**
  To allow for the integration and balance of the transformational energy awakened

- **Meditation**
  (Can be reversed with relaxation.) To support, seal and accelerate the development of pure conscious, awareness and experience of one's true identity – Sat Nam

- **Closing Blessing/Quote/Prayer**
  May the Long Time Sun Shine Upon You
  All Love Surround You
  And The Pure Light Within You
  Guide Your Way On
  Saaaaat Naaam
  Truth Is My Identity (used extensively in Kundalini practices and is both a greeting and a closing mantra)

  Kundalini Yoga is... a practice of experience of a person's own excellence which is dormant and then awakened

  - Yogi Bhajan 7/26/96

Experiencing Kundalini

I encourage you to seek the experience of Kundalini Yoga. Please use the resource guide at the end of this section to find classes near you or web-based information and practice. Below are two of my favorite Kundalini Meditations for your use and experience.

NowOpp@KundaliniMeditationForAddiction

For Healing Addictive Behavior

Sit in Easy Pose, with a light jalandhar bandh. Straighten the spine and make sure the first six lower vertebrae are locked forward.

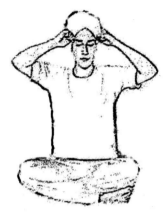

Eyes: Keep the eyes closed and focus at the Brow Point.

Mantra: SAA-TAA-NAA-MAA

Mudra: Make fists of both hands and extend the thumbs straight. Place the thumbs on the temples and find the niche where the thumbs just fit. This is the lower anterior portion of the frontal bone above the temporal-sphenoidal suture. Lock the back molars together and keep the lips closed. Keeping the teeth pressed together throughout, alternately squeeze the molars tightly and then release the pressure. A muscle will move in rhythm under the thumbs. Feel it massage the thumbs and apply a firm pressure with the hands. Silently vibrate the five primal sounds - the Panj Shabd - SAA-TAA-NAA-MAA, at the brow.

Time: Continue for 5-7 minutes. With practice, the time can be increased to 20 minutes and ultimately to 31 minutes.

Comments: This meditation is one of a class of meditations that will become well-known to the future medical society. Meditation will be used to alleviate all kinds of mental and physical afflictions. But it may be as many as 500 years, however, before the new medical science will understand the effects of this kind of meditation well enough to delineate and measure all its parameters. The pressure exerted by the thumbs triggers a rhythmic reflex current into the central brain. This current activates the brain area directly underneath the stern of the pineal gland. It is an imbalance in this area that makes mental and physical addictions seemingly unbreakable.

In modern culture, this imbalance is pandemic. If we are not addicted to smoking, eating, drinking, or drugs, then we are addicted subconsciously to acceptance, advancement, rejection, emotional love, etc. All of these lead us to insecure and neurotic behavior patterns. Imbalance in this pineal area upsets the radiance of the pineal gland itself. It is this pulsating radiance that regulates the pituitary gland. Since the pituitary regulates the rest of the glandular system, the entire body and mind go out of balance. This meditation corrects the problem. It is excellent for everyone but particularly effective for rehabilitation efforts in drug dependence, mental illness, and phobic conditions.

NowOpp@ KundaliniMeditationFor/Emotional Balance

Sunia(n) Antar

Before beginning this meditation drink a glass of water.

Sit in Easy Pose.

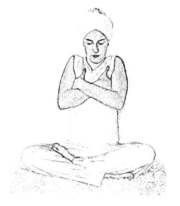

Mudra: Place the arms across the chest and lock hands under the armpits, with palms open and against the body. Raise the shoulders up tightly against the earlobes, without cramping the neck muscles. Apply Neck Lock.

Eyes: Close the eyes.

Breath: The breath will automatically become slow.

Time: Continue for three minutes, gradually increasing to 11 minutes.

Comments: This meditation is call Sunia(n) Antar. It is very good for women. It is essential at times when one is wounded or upset and doesn't know what to do, or when one feels like screaming, yelling, or misbehaving. When out of focus or emotional, attention should be given to the body's water balance and breath rate. Humans are approximately 70 percent water, and behavior depends upon the relation of water and earth, air and ether. Breath, representing air and ether, is the rhythm of life. Normally, we breathe 15 times a minute, but when we are able to rhythmically slow down the breath to only 4 breaths per minute, we have indirect control over our minds. This control eliminates obnoxious behavior, promoting a calm mind regardless of the state of affairs. When there is a water imbalance in the system, and the kidneys are under pressure, it can cause worry and upset. Drinking water, pulling the shoulders up to the ears and tightly locking the entire upper area creates a solid brake that can be applied to the four sides of the brain. After 2 or 3 minutes, thoughts will still be there, but one does not feel them. This is a very effective method of balancing the functional brain.

Kundalini Resource Guide:

International Kundalini Yoga Website – www.3ho.org
International Kundalini Research Institute – www.kriteachings.org
Kundalini Yoga for Addictive Behavior – http://super-health.net
Guru Ram Das Center for Medicine and Humanology – www.grdcenter.org
Teacher and Trainer Harijiwan Singh Kalsa - www.harijiwan.com
Kundalini Meditation: Guided Chakra Practices, by Harijiwan Singh Kalsa

Merging Rivers Retreats – www.mergingrivers.com

For CD's, DVD, and other Kundalini related things - www.spiritvoyage. com

The Aquarian Teacher, by Yogi Bhajan, Ph.D.

The Master's Touch, by Yogi Bhajan, Ph.D.

Kundalini Yoga Meditation for Psychiatric Disorders, Couples Therapy and Personal Growth, by David S. Shannahoff-Khalsa

The Psychospiritual Clinician's Handbook – Alternative Methods for Understanding and Treating Mental Disorders, by Sharon G. Mijares, Ph.D. and Gurucharan Singh Khalsa, Ph.D.

Meditations for Addictive Behavior - A system of Yoga Science and Nutritional Formulas, by Makta Kaur Khalsa, Ph.D.

Pranayama

Pranayama is a Sanskrit word derived from **prana**, which means *breath*, and **ayama,** which means *restraining* or *controlling, or expanding*. Some people call pranayama the yoga of breath.

> *The main problem in the world is stress.*
> *It is not going to decrease – it is going*
> *to increase. If through pranayam the*
> *shock can be harnessed, the entire*
> *disease of stress can be eliminated.*

-Yogi Bhajan, Ph.D., Kundalini Yoga Master

The vast healing system of Pranayam or conscious use of the breath is a wonderland of healing, awareness and expanded consciousness opportunities. The important thing to remember is this practice is not only learning how to breathe with our physical breathing features and system of respiration, but also with the subtle life force of the body called prana. Pranayam is the practice of connecting and communing with the very Life Force. It is a force that supplies all that we need for life, connection to all things, and introduces us to our infinite selves.

In the beginning, there was the word/breath/vibration/sound. These words have an intimate interrelatedness, and have been attributed to the power of the Source of all things and the language of God. The breath is foundational as the source of life and the vehicle for expression of thoughts, emotion, communication and relationship. Through the conscious use of the breath, we consciously co-create our lives.

The most complete and organized system of pranic healing in my opinion is included the Kundalini Yoga and Meditation Technology, and that is the structure I will follow for this chapter on Pranayam. The dual attention awareness of Kundalini teachings and many indigenous cultures offer the skills we need to truly understand and experience the healing practices optimally. Breath has this two-sided nature of the finite and the infinite. Pranayam interacts with all the aspects and nature of our existence and forms the matrix of our consciousness. It moves and affects all things. The breath is a healing tool, emotionally, physically, mentally and spiritually, for developing the ability of second awareness or second attention along with the practice of pranayam as a process of becoming your own healer.

The Many Benefits of Pranayam - Our Most Available and Powerful Tool of Transformation

- Promotes health and vitality at deep and high levels
- Stimulates creativity, solution-oriented thinking and lateral thinking
- Releases stuck emotion and deepens capacity for emotions
- Deepens the capacity for life on all levels
- Controls moods and balances the psyche
- Develops concentration and expanded brain function
- Opens the feeling of connection and clarity
- The mind follows the breath. To change the mind, change the breath
- Peace and stillness are found in a new rhythm of breath
- Every state of being has a breath signature. To change a state of being, change the breath

Some Basic Categories of Pranayam Technique

With that understanding, we will proceed with further knowledge about pranayam regarding some of the many techniques and their predictable effect when practiced.

1. Natural Breath - The Correct Normal Breath – for proper "unconscious" breathing technique
2. Breath Frequency – One Minute Breath – Dramatically calms anxiety, fear and worry/optimizes left and right brain hemispheres
3. Breath Length – Long Deep Breathing relaxes and calms/ stimulates the parasympathetic nervous system
4. Breath Suspension – Suspending the breath in or out - Reconditioning the Nervous System
5. Segmented Breath – Stimulates the Central Brain and Glandular System
6. Alternate Nostril Breath – Covers all stages of the pranayam practice
7. Emphasizing inhaling boosts the sympathetic part of the nervous system, prepares for action
8. Emphasizing exhaling stimulates the parasympathetic nervous system, prepares for relaxation and promotes elimination physically and emotionally

Cautions for Pranayam Practice

- Never force the breath. Be sensitive to the body.
- If dizziness occurs, stop and breath naturally until you rebalance.
- If you are on the first three days of the menstrual cycle or in first trimester pregnancy, refrain from breath of fire.
- Practice pranayam for only short periods of time. Do not overdo.

Pranayam – Breath Exercises and NowOpps

Breath is the essence of life. You inhale for the first time as you arrive in the world, and from that moment on, you take approximately

17,000 breaths each day, which over an average lifetime, totals about 500 million. Any attention to and consciousness of your breathing is a major step to a lifelong practice that can purify you, energize you, calm you and connect you at a very deep level. Here are some of the more well-known pranayam techniques. You can feel the results for yourself by treating each of them as a NowOpp. For all practices, consciously take note of your state of being for comparison after the practice.

Natural Breath – Relearning What You Knew as a Baby

Just watch a baby for a model of this breath. The navel point moves out on the inhale and in and up on the exhale. The inhale makes us wider and the exhale makes us longer. This usually seems backwards from the way we have unlearned to breath.

NowOpp@NaturalBreath

Practice the natural breath to get the feeling of the correct dynamic. This stimulates the brain and stimulates the pituitary and the third eye chakra.
Variation:

- Lengthen and exaggerate the inhale, and then do the same for the exhale for a cleansing breath

---

One-Minute Breath

On mastery of the one minute breath...
All knowledge of the universe, here and hereafter, of the
underworld and the heavenly skies, will dawn on you.

-Yogi Bhajan, Ph.D.

Benefits include optimized cooperation between the brain hemispheres, dramatic calming of anxiety, fear and worry, openness to feeling one's presence of Spirit. As intuition develops, the whole brain works better, especially the brain stem and frontal hemispheres.

NowOpp@OneMinuteBreath

The cycle of this breath is ultimately one minute in total - twenty second inhale, twenty second hold, and twenty second exhale. Caution: Begin very slowly with five to ten second segments and increase over time as is comfortable. Never force this breath. Consistent, gentle practice is the key to mastery.

- Be comfortable and still
- Take a few minutes to relax and deepen your breath
- Inhale slowly and steadily, filling your lower abdomen, your stomach area, up to your lungs and all the way up your chest
- Lock the breath once you filled your upper chest and hold
- Exhale, slowly and gently and steadily
- At the end of the exhale, gently reverse to an inhale

If you feel yourself struggling at any time, pause and do long deep breathing and begin again.

Nadi Shodhana - The Alternate Nostril Breathing Exercise:

Nadi Shodhana is a simple form of alternate nostril breathing suitable for beginning and advanced students. Nadi means "channel" and refers to the subtle energy pathways in the body through which prana flows. Shodhana means "cleansing" -- so Nadi Shodhana means channel cleansing or subtle energy channel purification.

Left nostril breathing only is associated with cooling, calmness, empathy, sensitivity and synthesis. Right nostril breathing is associated with vigor, alertness, willpower, concentration and readiness for action.

The benefits of alternate nostril breathing are a calmer mind, reduced stress and anxiety, and balances the left and right hemispheres, which promotes clear thinking. Just five minutes of it makes a big difference. It is a great way to prepare for meditation, or even when you are trying to fall asleep.

NowOpp@AlternateNostrilBreathing

Hold your right hand up and curl your index and middle fingers toward your palm. Place your thumb next to your right nostril and your ring finger and pinky by your left. Close the right nostril by pressing gently against it with your thumb, and inhale through the left nostril. The breath should be slow, steady and full. Now close the left nostril by pressing gently against it with your ring finger and pinky, and open your right nostril by relaxing your thumb and exhale fully with a slow and steady breath. Inhale through the right nostril, close it, and then exhale through the left nostril. That's one complete round of Nadi Shodhana. Keep going....

Inhale through the left nostrile- Exhale through the right
Inhale through the right nostril - Exhale through the left
Inhale through the left - Exhale through the right
Inhale through the right - Exhale through the left
Inhale through the left - Exhale through the right . . . . Etc....

Begin with 5-10 rounds and add more as you feel ready. Remember to keep your breathing slow, easy and full – you can do it for up to eleven minutes, but begin with three minutes.

You can do this just about any time and anywhere. Try it as a mental warm-up before meditation to help calm the mind and put you in the mood. Also, try it at times throughout the day. Nadi Shodhana helps control stress and anxiety. If you start to feel stressed out, ten or so rounds will help calm you down. It also helps soothe the temporary anxiety caused by air travel and other fearful or stressful situations.

Long Deep Yogic Breathing

Long deep breathing brings expanded aerobic capacity, cleansing, centering and relaxation of the nervous system. It counteracts the shallow rapid breaths that occur during the stress response. We may use only 600 cubic centimeters of our lung volume and we are capable of 6000. It is an easy preparation for meditation and yoga. This is the simplest and most natural of yogic breaths.

NowOpp@LongDeepYogicBreath

You can do this sitting up or even lying down.

Inhale slowly through the nostrils beginning with relaxing, filling the abdominal area first, then the chest cavity, then the clavicle area. Visualize expanding the body in 360 degrees as you inhale.

Once the lungs are completely filled in this manner, hold the breath lightly for a moment and press the shoulders back and expand the chest out so that the full length and pressure on the diaphragm can be felt.

Exhale slowly through the nostrils beginning with the clavicle area, then the chest cavity, and then the abdominal area, contracting your navel area to completely clear the lungs.

By breathing in this way through the nostrils for several breaths, the circulation in the diaphragm increases and the pressure in all areas of the lungs also generates stimulation and energy in all the nerve endings. The entire body is enlivened by the breath and the awakening of the nerves.

Long Deep Breathing is done using muscles of the abdomen, chest and shoulder areas and you can begin to feel the sensation of a natural bellows-like motion in the diaphragm.

Strive to extend the length of the inhale and exhale and have them equal in time.

Meaning, if your inhale takes seven seconds...exhale for seven seconds. Hold the breath for a count of one or two between the inhale and the exhale.

4/4 Breath for Energy

This breath will relax and energize you and help combat encroaching fatigue or emotion. In games or sports, it can rejuvenate coordination and spirit, and possibly help avoid injury. This is a great quick pickup when you have only a minute. If you do it two to three times a day at strategic times (before meals, meetings, driving home, etc.) and when you begin to feel tired, you will notice a big difference in the way you feel. Do it at 3:00 P.M. to avoid the 3:00 P.M. sinking syndrome.

NowOpp@SegmentedBreathFor Energy

Sit straight placing the palms together at the Heart Center with the fingers pointing up. Focus at the Brow Point with the eyelids lightly closed. Inhaling, break the breath into four equal segments, parts or sniffs, filling the lungs completely on the fourth breath. As you exhale, release the breath in four equal segments, completely emptying the lungs on the fourth breath. On each part of the inhale and exhale, pull in the navel point. The stronger you pump the navel, the more energy you will generate. One full breath cycle (in and out) takes about 7-8 seconds. Continue for two to three minutes. If you press the hands together very hard, and do it vigorously, one minute will recharge you and alter your mental state. If you are anxious or confused, add the mantra Sa Ta Na Ma mentally on both the inhale and the exhale.

To end, press the palms forcefully together for 10 to 15 seconds creating a tension in the whole body by pressing as hard as you can. Hold as long as possible. Exhale powerfully and repeat...Inhale, hold and exhale. Relax and feel all the tension in the body vanish. If you need rest, immediately lie on the back with the eyes closed and allow each area of the body to relax for two more minutes. Take a few deep breaths, stretch and you will be ready for action.

Breath of Fire

Breath of Fire is a cleansing and energizing breath powered by abdominal contractions. Once you become aware of the movement of the diaphragm during Long Deep Breathing, then you can easily do Breath of Fire. The air is pulled in and pumped out very rhythmically just like pumping a bellows without any tension being felt whatsoever on the abdominal muscles, chest and rib cage muscles. Your shoulders will remain relaxed throughout the breath, so that it may almost seem as though you can continue the rhythm indefinitely with little effort at all.

This breath brings activation of the energy system from the navel point, cleanses the lungs and oxygenates and purifies your blood stream. This instantly relieves stress and anxiety. It is used often in Kundalini Yoga.

NowOpp@BreathOfFire

Inhale and exhale with no pause through the nose in an equal rhythm. The exhale is activated at the navel point. Begin with a comfortable rhythm and increase speed as is comfortable. While breathing mentally, repeat Sat (rhymes with "but") on the inhale and Nam (rhymes with "Tom") on the exhale.

You can start with long deep breathing then, as soon as the lungs are completely expanded, as described earlier, immediately force the air out, and as soon as most of the air is out, immediately expand the air back in, each time arching the spine forward and pressing the palms inward against the knees in a light manner to feel the diaphragm filling the lungs from the back to the front completely, then contracting again. With each breath, one expands a bit faster and contracts a bit faster until, without expanding or contracting completely, a rhythm is felt, and you let that rhythm take over. You might liken it to an old model locomotive where the wheels lurch forward until some steam and speed is built up, then suddenly the train is moving forward almost effortlessly, with each breath like the chugging sound of the locomotive.

Breath of Fire will entirely charge the nervous system causing the glands to secrete and purify the blood. When it is done with certain postures and movements which are meant to put contracting (drawing in) or expanding (releasing) pressure in nerve plexuses and glandular centers, those areas are made to fire and become completely charged.

As this charge builds and polarizes, the mind becomes very still, very clear and bright, and radiance is felt in and through and around the body and head.

The feeling of the stressful need to think and act and to be the "doer," begins to recede as the mind becomes more receptive and open to noticing that there seems to be an almost automatic connectedness between one's aims and events and experiences that come to fulfill them. The feeling of a natural ever-present oneness begins to emerge as a clearer, always existing, reality.

4 -4 -2 Breath

When we experience fear and anxiety consciously or unconsciously, we tend to hold our breath. This signals your nervous system that you are in danger. The 4-4-2 breath helps to send a message to your nervous system letting it know that you are safe. This breath enables you to deal with the fear and anxiety in a more effective and healthy way.

NowOpp@442Breath

Inhale deeply to a slow count of four. Exhale immediately to a slow count of four. Then hold your breath for a slow count of two. Continue for at least five breaths.

Notice the change in the way you feel. This is a good breath to use at any time you wish to feel more relaxed and centered.

Sitali Pranayam

Sitali Pranayam is known to have a powerful cooling, relaxing effect on the body, while maintaining alertness. It is known to lower fevers, and aid digestion.

NowOpp@SitaliPranayam

- Curl the tongue into a "u" shape
- Inhale through the curled tongue
- Exhale through the nose.

You may notice the tongue tasting bitter at first. This is a sign of detoxification and will pass This breath is also used with Breath of Fire and with Segmented Breaths.

Pranayam Resource List

The Aquarian Teacher, by Yogi Bhajan, Ph.D.,
  Master of Kundalini Yoga
*Praana, Praanee, Praanayam, Exploring the Breath Technology of
  Kundalini Yoga as taught by Yogi Bhajan*®
Body, Mind, and Sport, by John Douillard
Breathing, Expanding your Power and Energy, by Michael Sky
*Soul Connection CD, Guided Meditations and Energy Healing for
  Extraordinary Health and Well Being,* by Andrea Becky Hanson

Section Seven

**Now Moment Mapping and
Planning Strategies**

Who Do You Think You Are Now?

For eons, we have been practicing being physical human beings, when we are actually spiritual human beings. We have some ground to make up. We need more practice being our true selves and navigating successfully with grace and ease, connected and in service to others without struggle and sacrifice in our new world. Now that you have a bit of a different image of who you are, why you are here, and what is important, work with the questions below and compare your answers to those at the front of the book.

NowApp@WhoYouAreNow

- Who are you?
- Where do you live?
- Why are you here?
- What laws do you live by?
- What keys are on your key ring?
- What languages do you speak?
- Who is on your life consulting team?

The Secrets of a Joyous Life:

My life is my message.

-Mahatma Ghandi

1. Know and experience yourself at the level of your Soul.
2. Be open to, know the value of, understand and be grateful for your unique gifts and talents.
3. Live your life purpose being present for whatever life offers. Remain open to the guidance of the Divine Source, and in the awareness of serving others using your unique gifts.
4. Consciously co-create your life story as a positive legacy with each thought, word and action, meaningful communication and relationship, and excellence on all levels.
5. Dare to live in excellence, humility, gratitude, compassion, forgiveness and connection to all things.

Your Round Table Consulting Team and Your Board of Advisors

The significant problems in our lives cannot be solved at the same level of understanding that we were at when they were created.

-Albert Einstein

At some stage, I realized that who was advising me were people and things from my past. They were either in person or in my conditioned mind and were involved with perpetuating the problems I was trying to solve! When I started replacing those advisors with advisors that had my better interests in mind, things started going a lot better. The chart on the next page will assist you with this process.

Select your consulting team from the aspects of you and the universal energies. This includes the keys and languages that are your bridge from the unseen to the seen and from the unmanifest to the manifest. It can include the archetypes...anything that attracts your attention that you want to inform you. You can also include spiritual beings, people that have passed over, guides, angels, etc. For an example, at my round table is usually intuition, the unknown, my heart, my skeptic, emotions...etc., and the Mother-Father God are permanent members of my consulting team. Each time you call a meeting, you can call in anything and anyone to assist you.

The board of advisors is slightly different. They are needed in very specific circumstances...like the rational mind for financial decisions, like saints and angels for spiritual matters and crises, maybe Mother Theresa... You get the idea. This is all playful and fun, but what it does is keep you aware of your complete connectedness and pure potentiality.

You can have regular meetings or just as needed. The bottom line is stay in touch with all that is and ask for what you need. Oh, and by the way, you can ask anyone or anything that has ill-advised you to leave...permanently.

Use the universal laws as guidelines for discussions and decisions. If you are trying to do something that is not compatible with the tenets of the universal laws. It will be a terrible waste of time and energy. Only 100% pure light and energy allowed. Consulting the universal laws in the process helps make life joyous and flow with grace and ease.

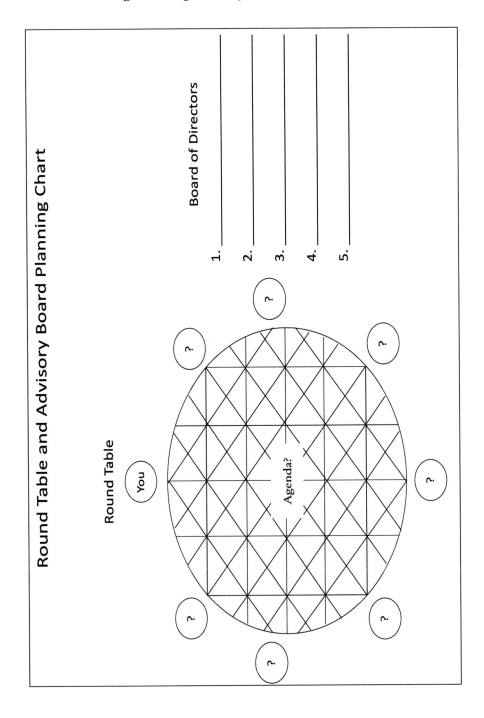

Round Table and Advisory Board Planning Chart

Board of Directors

1.

2.

3.

4.

5.

Round Table

You

?

?

?

?

?

?

?

Agenda?

Matrix Cluster Planning

*There are two ways to live your life.
One is as though nothing is a miracle.
The other is as though everything is a miracle.*

-Albert Einstein

What I have learned about personal plans for self realization is that the person seeking personal growth and spiritual evolution must design their own plan for it to be authentic and effective. In *Light Through the Keyhole* I have shared my experience of what I have found to be the best knowledge, awareness, understanding to heighten your awareness and your knowledge of yourself and holistic energy healing practices. With the Matrix Chart on the next page, begin to plan for your individual life practice.

What I recommend here is to use what I call "Matrix Cluster Planning." Avoid making lists of things to do. Begin by examining the Matrix Planning Resource Chart. It is a matrix of possibilities both from the past and future, and the keys and languages and techniques and therapies you are now aware of. As you look it over, feel into what appeals to you and what you are most interested in. This is a process for the creative mind.

Then go to Matrix Life Planning Chart Number Two. Again, examine the chart and decide how you want to organize your future plans regarding your personal practice. It could be organized into what you select for your spiritual practice or emotional, mental, physical and spiritual categories. It could be personal, family, career, social, environmental, and spiritual or, it could be specific areas like communication, relationship, abundance, etc., and/or any combination you choose. Use your unique imagination and the knowledge of what you most deeply desire and begin to place your plans and goals throughout the chart. This is best done in pencil and over time. Incorporate or activate what you choose in some way within twenty-four hours of placing it in the chart to ignite your plans and keep the transformational fires going.

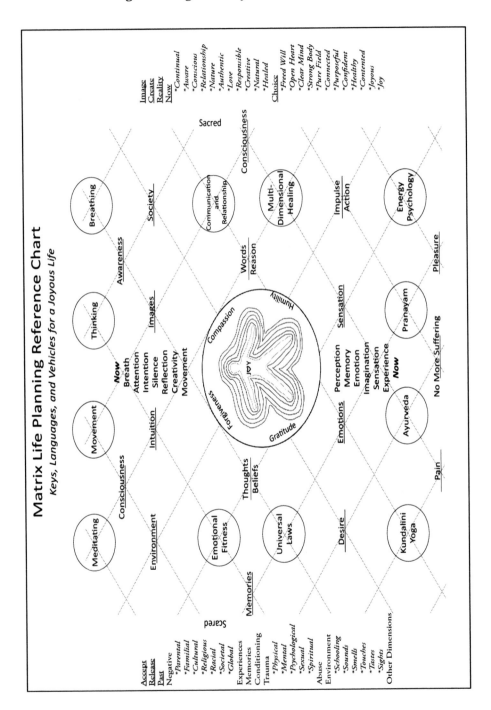

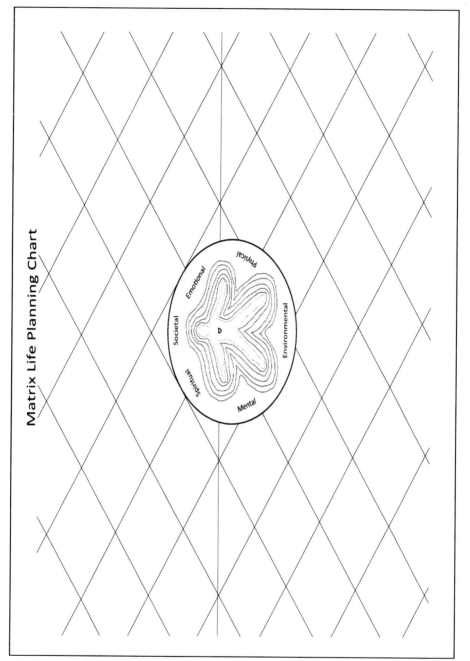

Master Matrix Life Planning Chart #2

An Overall Strategy for Planning a Personal Practice

1. Design, develop and implement a spiritual practice, including anything you found interesting and including some yoga, meditation, pranayam and Ayurvedic knowledge to make better choices.
2. Set a realistic and regular schedule for your practice and make it fun. Regular loving practice results in higher states of conscious awareness.
3. Tap, tap, tap...on everything, anytime, anywhere using the principle of attention and intention.
4. Feed your creative self, with awareness of creative opportunities, movement, journaling, creative visual meditation and studying new subjects.
5. Risk expressing your true feelings to accelerate the development of your authentic self as a state of being.
6. Avoid toxic people, places, foods and environments.
7. Consult with yourself via the C.I.A. (Check in and ask) meditation regularly, and consult with your round table advisors and advisory board regularly.
8. Review and renew your practice plans as you evolve and feel the need.
9. Don't make your spiritual practice a guilt trip. Be kind and gentle with yourself.
10. Use *Light Through the Keyhole* as a reference, and stay in touch: www.mergingrivers.com www/facebook.com/MergingRiversHealingPractices

Sat Nam!

Andrea Becky

Andrea Becky's Closing Message

Dear Reader

Dare to be honestly vulnerable, deeply connected with others, and live a joyous life.

It has been my honor and pleasure to share what I have learned with you. Thank you.

From my heart and soul, I hope this book has informed and inspired you, and changed your life in ways that you desired.

I wish you all your deepest driving desires manifested, and your direct experience and realization of your true excellence and joy.

Sat Nam

Andrea Becky

Section Eight

Glossary, Additional Resources and Support Material

Glossary of Holistic Energy Healing Terms

1. **Acupoint:** Point of least resistance along a meridian used for treatment
2. **Ahimsa:** Non-injury, non-violence, harmlessness
3. **Asanas:** Yoga Postures or movements with specific intention for health and meditation
4. **Ashram:** Retreat or secluded place, usually where the principles of yoga and meditation are taught and practiced
5. **Belief Gap:** The distance between a new concept and current perception
6. **Bhakti Yoga:** The yoga path of love and devotion
7. **Biofield:** The total human field of energy and information
8. **Brahman:** The absolute divinity itself
9. **Breath:** Universal life force that permeates all things
10. **Buddhi:** The discerning intellect
11. **Chakras:** Sanskrit for "wheel" or living energy centers within the human field processing the life force (Chi, Prana, Qi, Manna, etc.) energy and information. There are eight major centers "located" along the spine from the base to the crown and above
12. **Chi:** Chinese word for universal life energy force
13. **Choice Point:** The point of decision that changes a current situation
14. **Contemplation/Dhyana:** The meditative practice of consciously contemplating possibilities which is calming to the mind
15. **Cymatics:** The study of the effect of sound on matter
16. **Dharana:** Concentration or holding the mind in one thought
17. **Dharma:** Self-discipline, the life of responsibility and right action of the higher Self
18. **Dhyana:** Deep meditation
19. **Dosha:** Elements making up mind/body composition
20. **Electophotonic Capture:** A method of measuring energy fields, states of being and Consciousness
21. **Electrobiomagnetic Microscopes:** Capable of seeing the tiny forms of matter and how it behaves
22. **Energy Healing:** Discovering and harmonizing living energies, known and unknown, on all levels, intellectual, physical, emotional and spiritual

23. **Energy Medicine:** A body of knowledge offering alternative natural treatments and therapies for healing based on the holistic approach to healing and well-being
24. **Energy Psychology:** The process by which self-defeating patterns can be deconstructed and replaced with a sense of true self, higher levels of psychological, physical, spiritual and emotional well-being and overall joy of being, and can be maintained effortlessly
25. **Eternal Now Moment:** The only real time
26. **Felt Sense:** A sense of knowing that is felt in the body or senses
27. **Guna:** The three major Gunas: sattva (preservation), rajas (creation), and tamas (destruction), are the operating principles of life and carry out the process of life. Guna itself, means string or thread in Sanskrit
28. **Grounding and Centering:** The process of centering within the human field
29. **Hatha Yoga:** Master of the polarities. It is the yoga of physical well-being, designed to balance body, mind, and spirit
30. **Holistic Healing:** Healing that is based on the whole organism, balance and harmony
31. **Holo-energetic Healing:** Healing with the energy of the whole
32. **Informational Substances:** Molecules (ligands) that carry chemical information to the cells. They can act on their own cell, on cells nearby, or at large distances in the body
33. **Japa Yoga:** The path of mantra recitation
34. **Kirlian Phototography:** Photographing the heat of energy fields
35. **Kundalini Energy:** The dominant spiral or "coiled snake." Energy dormant within the base chakra waiting to be awakened, raised and distributed and balanced within the human field
36. **Kundalini Mantra Meanings**
    a. Sa Ta Na Ma – Infinity, Life, Death, Rebirth – Cycle of Creation and Healing
    b. Sat Nam – True Identity
    c. Wahe Guru – Ecstasy of Indescribable Wisdom
    d. Ong Namo Guru Dayv Namo – I bow to the subtle divine wisdom
    e. Har (Hud) – The Creative Infinity of God

37. **Kundalini Yoga:** A yoga for the new millennia which corrects and balances the human energy field through stimulation of chakras, meridians, glands and central nervous system, on a cellular level. It is a Raj Yoga, complete in that it has retained the full round of yoga using asanas, pranayam, mantra/sound, music, and meditation, and provides a direct link to Awareness

38. **Ligand:** Any one of the family of information-bearing molecules in the body

39. **Mandala:** A circular geometric design that the represents the cosmos

40. **Matrix Learning: The ability to learn and experience information in a way that is not linear, and make later associations that bring understanding**

41. **Mantra:** Sound that has a healing, energetic effect on the human field

42. **Meditation** Technique: Directing attention and awareness. The discipline or practice of training the mind for neutral observance and healing the field. This inner-awareness allows us to be tranquil and move freely and effortlessly within the field with knowingness and awareness of the universal field of consciousness, all possibilities and potential

43. **Meditation:** The discipline or practice of training the mind for neutral observance and healing the field

44. **Meridian Therapies:** The technique of causing motion in the energy body's meridians in order to disperse blocks in the system

45. **Mudras:** Specific positions of the eyes and/or hands that create an energetic effect on the human energy field

46. **Muscle Testing:** Testing the resistance in particular indicator muscles to determine the human energy field's response to questions and information

47. **Myaya:** Rules, logic and rhetoric

48. **Namaste:** Hindu salutation meaning the divine in me honors the divine in you, and when we are both in that place, we are one. Often used upon meeting or parting and usually is accompanied by the gesture of holding the palms together in front of the heart. Pronounced NUM – ah – stay

49. **Neuroplasticity:** The scientific finding that the brain can change itself and its neuropathways
50. **Niyama:** Five disciplines (purity, contentment, purification, study, devotion)
51. **Neurotransmitters:** Simple molecules created by the brain to carry information across the synapses (gaps between neurons). Act more like hormones on receptors
52. **NowOpp:** Opportunity for immediate practice of a new concept or technique
53. **Not Having to Know:** Suspending need to know in order to get the greater meaning
54. **Om or Aum:** Mantras that represent the vibration of the universal field
55. **Ong:** Mantra that represents the pranic energy and focus within the human field
56. **Prana:** East Indian word for universal life energy force
57. **Pangea:** A united state of parts
58. **Pranayam:** The practice of conscious breathing for healing and integration
59. **Pranayam:** Control of prana (life Force)
60. **Pratyahar:** Synchronization of senses and thought
61. **Purva-Mimamsa:** Individual responsibility for one's actions and free will to create quality of life
62. **Psychosomatic Network:** The system of the body that mediates total health
63. **Qi:** Japanese word for universal life energy force
64. **Quantum Physics:** The science dealing with the smallest particles of life-revealing consciousness and an encompassing cosmic principle of Power and Love
65. **Raj Yoga:** The direct link to awareness, the Maha or greatest yoga
66. **Remote Healing:** Healing or viewing at a distance virtually.
67. **Resonant Healing:** Creating a very high frequency of healing energy
68. **Sadhana:** A spiritual devotional practice
69. **Samkhya:** Evolution of existence, nature of being, mental discrimination for perception of reality, rather than knowing through meditation

70. **Spiritual Beingness:** The state of being in a spiritual energy, while in the a physical body
71. **Spiritual Psychology:** The energetic vibrational approach to psychological, physical, intellectual, spiritual and emotional health
72. **String Theory:** The theory that has application to all things as being one
73. **Sutra:** A word or phrase that has deep and complex meaning
74. **Unified Field:** The entirety of all that is
75. **Vaisheshika:** Liberation by understanding all of existence in terms of these six primary categories
76. **Vedanta:** Internal experience and the nature of meditation, the mystic scriptures and integrated right action with the Oneness of creation and the nature of transcendental reality
77. **Yama:** Five restraints (non-hurting, truthfulness, non-stealing, sensory control, non-possessiveness)
78. **Yoga:** Practical techniques of meditation and self-control to attain the perception of self and reality, experiential learning

Additional Reading Resources

1. *Adrenal Fatigue,* by James L. Wilson, N.D., D.C., Ph.D.
2. *A Magnificent Mind at Any Age,* by Daniel G. Amen, M.D.
3. *Anastasia The Series,* by Vladimir Megré
4. *A Practical Guide to Vibrational Medicine,* by Richard Gerber, M.D.
5. *Art and Yoga,* by Hari Kirin Kaur Khalsa
6. *Cancer As Initiation - Surviving the Fire,* by Barbara Stone, Ph.D.
7. *Change Your Brain; Change Your Life,* by Daniel G. Amen, M.D.
8. *Energy Medicine,* by Donna Eden
9. *Esoteric Anatomy,* by Bruce Burger
10. *Hands of Light,* by Barbara Ann Brennan
11. *Invisible Roots,* by Barbara Stone, Ph.D., DEHP
12. *Light Emerging,* by Barbara Ann Brennan
13. *Love, The Real Da Vinci Code,* by Leonard G. Horowitz, D.D.S., Ph.D.
14. *Loving What Is,* by Byron Katie
15. *Many Minds, Many Masters,* by Brian L. Weiss, M.D.
16. *Matrix Energetics,* by Richard Bartlett, D.C., N.D.
17. *Molecules of Emotion,* by Candace Pert, Ph.D.
18. *Poems from the Edge of a New Reality,* by Andrea Becky Hanson
19. *Praana, Praanee, Praanayam, Technology of Kundalini Yoga,* by Yogi Bhajan, Ph.D.
20. *Quantum Health,* by Deepak Chopra, M.D.
21. *Right Use of Will, The Series,* by Ceanne DeRohan
22. *Sacred Mirrors,* by Alex Grey
23. *Soul Connection CD,* by Andrea Becky Hanson
24. *Spiritual Solutions,* by Deepak Chopra, M.D.
25. *The 5 Love Languages,* by Gary Chapman
26. *The Artist's Way,* by Julia Cameron
27. *The Complete Book of Water Therapy,* by Diane Buchman
28. *The Highest Level of Enlightenment,* by Dr. David Hawkins
29. *The Holographic Universe,* by Michael Talbot
30. *The Mind,* by Yogi Bhajan, Ph.D.
31. *The Promise of Energy Psychology,* by Feinstein, Eden and Craig

32. *The Soul of Leadership,* by Deepak Chopra, M.D.
33. *The Ten Light Bodies of Consciousness,* by Nirvair Singh Khalsa
34. *The War of World Views,* by Deepak Chopra M.D.
35. *Too Good to Leave, Too Bad to Stay,* by Mira Kirshenbaum
36. *Your Body Can Talk,* by Levy and Lehr
37. *Your Body Doesn't Lie,* by John Diamond, M.D.
38. *Your Body is Your Subconscious Mind,* Audiobook by Candace Pert, Ph.D.

Now/Opp@EnergyBalancingExercises
From Donna Eden's Amazing Comprehensive Book -
Energy Medicine

1. Zip Up

Feel more confident and positive.
Be more present with other people.
Tap your inner strengths.
Shield yourself from negative energies
With your intention, or using your hand, zip up from the pelvic floor
to under the lips.

2. Wayne Cook Posture

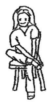

Untangle inner chaos. See with better perspective.
Focus your mind more effectively.
Think more clearly/take in info.
Learn more proficiently.
Hold the ankle of the crossed leg with the opposite hand. With the
same hand as the crossed leg, reach across and grasp the ball
of the foot. Breathe deeply and pull gently up and use a rocking
motion in that position. Repeat on the other side.
Uncross the legs. Then place finger and thumb tips together and
place thumb tips on lower center of forehead. Breathe deeply
and exhale slowly as you press lightly and pull thumb tips away
from each other towards the temples. Bring thumbs back to
forehead and then move hands to prayer pose, rest and breathe
deeply.

3. Three Thumps

Energize if feeling drowsy.
Focus if having difficulty concentrating.
Increase vitality.
Keeps immune system strong amid stress.
Tap or massage the points indicated (just under the collar bone, center of the chest, lower front ribs). Tap or three to five times with the fingers of either or both hands. Breathe deeply and relax.

4. Cross Crawl

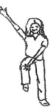

Feel more balanced. Crosses right and left brain.
Think more clearly.
Improves coordination.
Harmonizes your energies.
Promotes healing.
Lift opposite leg and arm to touch knee going from side to side. It is like an exaggerated march. Continue for at least one minute. You can add counting if you wish, one to 20 and/or backwards from 20 to one, hum, or do the alphabet.

5. Heaven and Earth

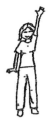

Activates respiratory system. Pulls in extra oxygen to cells. Releases carbon dioxide.

Opens joints. Releases trapped energy.

Start with hands at your side. Inhale through the nose and circle arms up and bring hands to prayer pose at chest level.

Exhale through mouth. Inhale through nose and separate hands with one palm facing heaven and one facing earth and hold as long as possible. Exhale through the mouth. Return your hands to prayer pose. Repeat the sequence changing the arm that raises. When you come out of the pose, allow yourself to fold over at the waist and hang there with knees slightly bent for two deep breaths. Slowly return to standing position and roll shoulders back and down.

6. Crown Pull

Releases mental congestion. Refreshes the mind.

Opens crown chakra to higher inspiration.

Often relieves headache.

Place thumbs on the temples and fingertips on forehead just above the eyebrows. With light pressure, pull your finger tips apart across your forehead. Moving your fingertips up and back slightly each time you repeat the motion moving all the way to the back over your head to the back of the head. Repeat each of these stretches one or more times.

7. Spinal Flush

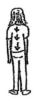

Cleanses lymphatic system. Stimulates cerebrospinal fluid.
Clears stagnant energies.
Send toxins to body's waste removal system.
Immediately takes edge off emotional overreactions.
Do at first symptoms of a cold.
You may lie face down or stand supporting yourself against a wall.
  Have a partner massage each side of your spine between the
  notches of your vertebrae for about five seconds from neck to
  sacrum. Then with an open hand and a sweeping motion from the
  shoulders to the heels, sweep the energies down your body and
  off your feet two to three times.

Additional Resources

Kundalini Yoga Mantras and Meaning
TUNE IN MANTRA
Ong Namo Guru Dev Namo
(Creator) (Reverernt Greetings) (Darkness to Light) (Non-Physical) (Reverent Greetings)

I bow to (call on) the infinite power of the universe, the divine teacher within.

MANGALA CHARAN MANTRA
Aad Guray Nameh
I call the primal wisdom

Jugaad Guray Nameh
I call to the wisdom of the ages

Sat Gudey Nameheh
I bow to the true wisdom

Siree Guroo Day Va Nameh
I call upon the transparent wisdom within

This mantra is used for centering and protection.

LONG TIME SUN BLESSING FOR THE SELF,
LOVED ONES, AND ALL BEINGS
May the Long Time Sun Shine Upon You
All Love Surround You
And the Pure Light Within You
Guide Your Way On
Guide Your Way On

GREETING AND CLOSING
Saaaat Naam
Tuth is my identity
We are Truth

AHHH KAAAL
Ahhh Kaaaal
Undying... Used to connect and support a departed soul in making the transition through the layers that bind the spirit to this dimension. Especially for 17 days after death. Helpful in healing grief.

LAYA YOGA MEDITATION
Ek Ong Kaar (Uh)
(The creator and All Creation Are One)
Sa Ta Na Ma (Uh)
(Infinity, Birth, Death, Rebirth - Cycle of All Creation)
Siree Wha (Uh)
The Ecstasy of This Wisdom)
Hay Guroo
(Is Great Beyond Words)

The rhythm of this chant gives it a "spinning energy." It rotates the energy of all the chakras and the aura, integrating your energy, creativity, focus, and discernment.

AAD SACH (BHAY VERSION)
Aad Sach jugaad sach, hai bhay sach,
True in the beginning, True throughout the ages, True at this moment
Naanak hose bhay sach
Truth shall be forever

Connects the speaker to the infinite and the infinite to the speaker.

GURU MANTRA OF GURU RAM DAS
Guru Guru Wahe Guru
Teacher of Ecstasy of Light Wisdom
Guru Ram Das Guru
Teacher of healing the heart of the world

This chant energizes, balances and heals the entire field and assists in living in the Aquarian Age

SIRI MANTRA
Sa Ta Na Ma
Ra Ma Da Sa
Sa Say So Hung
SA/Infinity TA/Life NA/Death MA/Rebirth
RA/Sun MA/Moon DA/Earth SA/Infinity
SA/Infinity SAY/Thou HUNG/I am Thou

This is the most powerful mantra for healing on all levels taught to use for self or other

Note: For pronunciation and practice technique, refer to:
www.spiritvoyage.com; www.kundaliniresearchinstitute.org

Emotions and Emotional States of Being Reference Chart

Abandon	Abandoned	Above reproach	Abrasive	Abundant	Abundant
Abused	Accepting	Accused	Adventurous	Afraid	Ageless
Aggressive	Alert	Alive	Aloof	Anger	Anguished
Annoyed	Anticipate	Anxious	Apathy	Appreciative	Apprehensive
Argumentative	Arrogance	Arrogant	Ashamed	Assured	Aware
Awareness	Balance	Beautiful	Being	Belligerent	Belonging
Betrayed	Bigoted	Bliss	Blue	Boastful	Boiling
Bored	Bored	Boundless	Bright	Brooding	Caged
Callous	Calm	Can't wait	Can't win	Careless	Caustic
Cautious	Centered	Centered	Certain	Cheated	Cheerful
Childlike	Clammy	Clarity	Clever	Closed	Cold
Cold	Compassion	Compassionate	Competent	Complacent	Complete
Compulsive	Conceited	Condescending	Confident	Considerate	Constantly Recreated
Contemptuous	Courageousness	Cowardice	Craving	Creative	Critical
Cut-off	Daring	Dead	Decisive	Defeated	Defensive
Defiant	Delightful	Delusional	Demanding	Demanding	Demoralized
Depressed	Desolate	Despair	Despair	Destructive	Devious
Disappointed	Discouraged	Disdain	Disgust	Disillusioned	Distraught
Distrust	Divine Love	Divine Vibration	Dogmatic	Doomed	Doubt
Drained	Dread	Driven	Dynamic	Eager	Elated
Embarrassed	Embarrassed	Embracing	Empathy	Enriched	Enthusiastic
Envy	Eternal	Evasive	Everything's okay	Everywhere	Evolutionary

Emotions and Emotional States of Being Reference Chart

Exclusive	Exhilaration	Exploitative	Explorative	Explosive	Failure
Fair	False dignity	False Humility	False virtue	Fear	Fierce
Fixated	Flexible	Focused	Foreboding	Forgetful	Forgotten
Frantic	Free	Frenzy	Friendly	Frozen	Frustrated
Frustrated	Fulfilled	Fullness	Fully Awake	Fuming	Furious
Futile	Gentle	Get Even	Giving	Giving up	Gloating
Glowing	Glowing	Gluttonous	Gracious	Greedy	Grief
Guilty	Hardened	Harmonious	Harmony	Harsh'	Hate
Hatful	Haughty	Heartache	Heart-broken	Heartsick	Held Down
Helpless	Hesitant	Hoarding	Holier than thou	Honorable	Hopeless
Horrified	Hostility	Humor	Humorless	Hunger	Hurt
Hypocritical	Hysterical	I can	I can't	I don't care	I don't count
I have to have	I want	Icy	If only	Ignored	Immortal
Impatience	Impatient	In Gratitude	In tune	Inadequate	Inattentive
Inconsolable	Indecisive	Independent	Indifferent	Indignant	Infinite
Infinite Harmony	Infinite Organizing Power	Infinite Potential	Infinitely Creative	Inhibited	Initiative
Insecure	Integrity	Intricately connected	Intuitive	Invincible	Invisible
Irate	Irrational	It's all good	It's not fair	It's too late	Jealously
Joyful	Judgmental	Just	Know-it-all	Lascivious	Lazy
Lecherous	Left out	Let it wait	Light	Limitless	List
Listless	Livid	Longing	Longing	Loser	Loss

249

Lost	Loving	Loving	Lucid	Mad	Magnanimous
Manipulative	Mean	Melancholy	Mellow	Merciless	Miserly
Misunderstood	Motivated	Mourning	Murderous	Must have it	Narrow-minded
Naturalness	Nausea	Negative Numb	Neglected	Nervous	Never enough
Never satisfied	Never wrong	Nobody cares	Non-resistant	Nostalgia	Nostalgic
Nothing to change	Nourishing	Oblivious	Obsessed	Oneness	Open
Open	Opinionated	Optimistic	Outraged	Overbearing	Over-indulgent
Overwhelmed	Panic	Paralyzed	Paranoia	Passed over	Patronizing
Perfection	Perfectly Balanced	Perfectly Coherent	Perfectly Ordered	Perfectly Whole	Perspective
Petulant	Pious	Pity Poor me	Playful	Positive	Positive
Possessed	Possessive	Powerless	Predatory	Prejudiced	Presumptuous
Pure	Pure Knowledge	Pure Silence	Pushy	Pushy	Radiant
Rage	Raging	Rebellious	Receptive	Reckless	Regret
Rejected	Remorse	Resentment	Resentment	Resigned	Resilient
Resistant	Resourceful	Responsive	Revolted	Righteous	Rigid
Rude	Ruthless	Sadness	Savage	Scared	Scheming
Secretive	Secure	Secure	Self absorbed	Self satisfied	Selfish
Selfish	Self-Sufficient	Serenity	Settling	Shaky	Sharp
Shock	Shy	Silence	Simmering	Sizzling	Skeptical
Smoldering	Smothered	Smug	Snobbish	Soft	Sorrow
Space	Special	Spiteful	Spoiled	Spontaneous	Stage fright
Steely	Stern	Stewing	Still	Stoic	Stoned
Strong	Stubborn	Stubborn	Stuck	Stuck-up Superior	Sullen Vengeful

Emotions and Emotional States of Being Reference Chart

Superstitious	Suppressed	Suspicious	Tearful	Tender	Tense
Terrified	Territorial	Thankful	Threatened	Tied Down	Timeless
Timid	Tireless	Too tired	Tormented	Torn	Tortured
Total Health	Tranquil	Trapped	True Identity	Unbounded	Uncertain
Uncompromising	Understanding	Uneasy	Unfeeling	Unfeeling	Unfocused
Unforgiving	Unhappy	Unlimited	Unloved	Unwanted	Unyielding
Useless	Vague	Vain	Vicious	Vigorous	Vindictive
Violent	Visionary	Volcanic	Voracious	Vulnerable	Vulnerable
Want to escape	Wanton	Warm	Wary	Wasted	Well-being
What's the use?	Whole	Why me?	Why try?	Wicked	Wicked
Willing	Wonder	Worry	Worthless	Wounded	Youthful

Ishnan –The science of hydrotherapeutic massage.

"Ishnan" means the body itself creates the temperature that overcomes the coldness of water. It is done with great respect and grace towards the body. Those who practice this cross cultural healing method throughout the world, make many positive claims about the practice and its extraordinary benefits. Some of the healing benefits are:

- Keeps skin radiant
- Opens capillaries
- Flushes organs
- Keeps blood chemistry young and healthy
- Stimulates the healthy secretion of the glandular system.
- Strengthens the immune system.
- Balances metabolism

Now/Opp@Ishnan

Ishnan is a specific and precise science. Here are the steps and some of the effects of the process. The recommended duration of time is from three to five minutes

1. Dry brush the body with a natural bristle brush brushing towards the heart
2. Rub almond oil with long strokes on the long muscles and circular motion over all joints and the head.
3. Start a cold shower – Move into the cold water putting the extremities, feet, hands and arms under the water first and use either foot to massage the other. You need not use hands.
4. Cold Water on the face eliminates sleepiness, charges the energy and enhances clarity.
5. Cold Water on the front of the neck totally assists all your cells
6. Cold Water on the shoulders charges body chemistry
7. Cold Water on the upper arms heals the stomach
8. Cold Water on the lower arms heals the digestive system

---

9. Cold Water on the wrists heals the heart and liver
10. Cold Water on the backs of the thighs stimulates the brain

Precautions please:

- Thighs should not go under the water first
- Same for genitals and head
- Do not take cold showers during pregnancy or menstruation or with a fever, rheumatism or heart disease.
- If you have sciatic nerve or high blood pressure, start slowly.
- You can wear cotton shorts to protect and buffer the thighs and sexual organs.

Message to contemplate from the Hopi Elders, sages of our times.

Where are you living?
What are you doing?
What are your relationships?
Are you in right relation?
Where is your water?

Know your garden.
It is time to speak your Truth.
Create your community.
Be good to each other.
And do not look outside yourself for the leader.

This could be a good time! There is a river flowing now very fast. It is so great and swift that there are those who will be afraid. They will try to hold on to the shore. They will feel they are being torn apart and will suffer greatly.

Know the river has its destination.

The elders say we must let go of the shore, push off into the middle of the river, keep our eyes open, and our heads above the water.

See who is in there with you and celebrate.

At this time in history, we are to take nothing personally. Least of all, ourselves. For the moment that we do, our spiritual growth and journey comes to a halt.

The time of the lone wolf is over. Gather yourselves!

Banish the word struggle from your attitude and your vocabulary. All that we do now must be done in a sacred manner and in celebration.

We are the ones we've been waiting for.

Hopi Nation

Oraibi, Arizona

Live with Humility and only in Gratitude, Compassion, Forgiveness and Love... beginning with Self First.

-Andrea Becky Hanson 2011